MATH
FOR MEDS
DOSAGES AND SOLUTIONS

MATH
FOR MEDS
SIXTH EDITION
DOSAGES AND SOLUTIONS

Anna M. Curren

R.N. Royal Victoria Hospital, Montreal, PQ; B.N.
Dalhousie University, Halifax, Nova Scotia; M.A.
California State University, Long Beach, Calif.;
Former Associate Professor of Nursing, Long Beach
City College, Long Beach, Calif.

Laurie D. Munday

R.N. Los Angeles County U.S.C. Medical Center;
B.N. California State University, Los Angeles,
Calif.; M.N., C.S., U.C.L.A. Los Angeles, Calif.,
Former Assistant Professor of Nursing, San Diego
City College, San Diego, Calif.

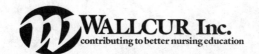
WALLCUR Inc.
contributing to better nursing education

ACKNOWLEDGEMENTS   Our first thank you must go to the hundreds of nurse educators who completed and returned evaluations of *Math For Meds*. These provided the direction for all changes implemented in the sixth edition. For allowing us to update in their clinical facilities in San Diego we especially thank Verna Nickel and the staff of Veterans Administration Hospital; Pat Keegan and the staff of Sharp Memorial Hospital; Marlene Ruiz and the staff of Kaiser Permanente Hospital; and Mary Ann Brainey and the clinical nursing specialists of Childrens Hospital. For assistance with the pediatric section we acknowledge the invaluable contribution of Shirley Naret, M.S.N., Ed.D., Professor of Nursing, Long Beach City College, Long Beach, Calif. Special thanks to David Onosko of IVAC Corporation for technical information, photos, and equipment loans.

The permission of the following companies and medical centers to reproduce medication labels and records, IV package labels, and syringe calibrations is gratefully acknowledged: Eli Lilly & Co.; Searle & Co,; Pharmacia Inc.; Ascot Pharmaceuticals; Lederele Laboratories; The William S. Merrell Company; Schering Pharmaceutical Corp.; Invenex; A.H. Robins Co.; Beecham Laboratories; Hoechst-Roussel Pharmaceuticals; J.B. Roerig; Merck, Sharp & Dohme; Smith, Kline & French Laboratories; The Upjohn Company; Mead Johnson & Company; Berlex Laboratories; Wyeth Laboratories, Inc.; Abbott Laboratories; Travenol Laboratories; Lyphomed, Inc.; Elkins-Sinn, Inc.; Glaxo Inc.; Cutter Laboratories; Becton Dickinson & Co. Ltd.; Toronto General Hospital; Lionville Systems, Inc.; and the University of California Medical Center, San Diego.

Printed in the United States of America

Library of Congress catalog card number 76-43259

Wallcur Inc.
3287 F Street, Suite G
San Diego, CA 92102
619-233-9628

Canadian Distributor
Login Brothers
Chicago, IL   Twinsburg, OH   Fairfield, NJ

PREFACE

The current sixth edition of *Math For Meds* continues to exemplify the very best learning format and instructional design in the area of dosages and solutions. Numerous illustrations, drug labels, hypodermic syringes and medication records function to provide a clinical reality unique to this subject area.

An increased need for basic math skills at all entry levels has mandated expansion of the refresher math section. Hundreds of examples and problems have been added to the instructional content offering the student an opportunity to excel in this area. All sections of the text have been revised and updated and overall content has been significantly increased.

An entirely new chapter on insulin calculations, combining dosages, and measurement with illustrated syringes has been added. Extensive revision of chapters relating to IV administration and flow rate calculation covers the most up to date drugs, and instructs each student with an easy to use step by step approach. Students are encouraged to work through the text at their own pace.

A totally revised section on pediatric medications includes oral, parenteral and IV calculation based on mg/kg and BSA. In-depth content on pediatric IV medication administration appears for the first time.

The comprehesive section on critical care enables students to work through a variety of complex but realistic problems and calculations before encountering them in the clinical area.

A choice of ratio and proportion or the formula method, the acknowledged safest methods of drug calculation, is offered throughout the text, with over 1500 problems ensuring mastery of every section. Comprehensive summary self tests follow each chapter allowing on-going testing of previously covered subject matter.

Content has been structured to meet all levels of nursing education, allied health, refresher and inservice programs. Extensive indexing allows instant retrieval of information, making *Math For Meds* an excellent resource for all health professionals.

Laurie D. Munday
Anna M. Curren
San Diego, Calif.

CONTENTS

SECTION
ONE
Refresher Math

1
Relative Value, Addition, and Subtraction of Decimals

OBJECTIVES
The student will
1. identify the relative value of decimals
2. add decimals
3. subtract decimals

PREREQUISITE
Recognize the abbreviation mg, for milligram, as a drug measure.

INTRODUCTION
In the course of administering medications you will be calculating drug dosages which contain decimals, for example 2.5 mg. The math you will need for these calculations is not difficult, and the first two chapters of this text will provide a complete and easy refresher of everything that you must know about decimals. Let's begin with a review of the relative value of decimals, so that you will be able to recognize which of two or more numbers has the highest (and lowest) value.

• RELATIVE VALUE OF DECIMALS •

The easiest way to begin a review of decimal numbers is to visualize them on a scale which has a decimal point at its center. Look for a moment at figure 1.

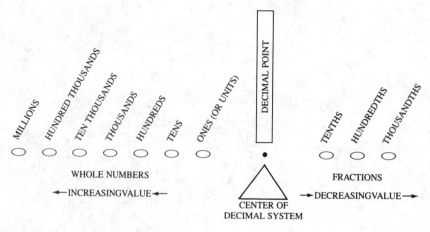

Figure 1

Notice that on the left of the decimal point are the whole numbers, and on the right the fractions. On the whole number (left) side of the scale the measures rise increasingly in value, from ones, to tens, to hundreds, and so on to millions, which is the highest measure you will see in drug dosages. Our monetary system of dollars and cents is a decimal system, and the relative value of the whole numbers is exactly as you now know and use them: the higher the number, the higher the value. Therefore, if a decimal number contains a whole number then the value of the whole number is the first determiner of relative value.

EXAMPLE 1   10.1 is higher than 9.1

EXAMPLE 2   3.2 is higher than 2.9

EXAMPLE 3   7.01 is higher than 6.99

PROBLEM

Identify the number with the highest value in each of the following.

> **1.** a) 3.5   b) 2.7   c) 4.2
>
> **2.** a) 6.15   b) 5.95   c) 4.54
>
> **3.** a) 12.02   b) 10.19   c) 11.04

ANSWERS   **1.** c   **2.** a   **3.** a

If, however, the whole numbers are the same, for example **10.**2 and **10.**7, or there are no whole numbers, for example **0.**25 and **0.**35, then the fraction will determine the relative value. Let's take a closer look at the fractional side of the scale. Refer to figure 2.

TENTHS   HUNDREDTHS   THOUSANDTHS

0   .   1   2   5

Figure 2

It is necessary to consider only three figures after the decimal point on the fractional side because drug dosages measured as decimal fractions do not contain more than three digits, for example 0.125 mg. First notice that **if a decimal fraction is not preceded by a whole number, a zero is used in front of the decimal point to emphasize that the number is a fraction**; for example 0.125, 0.1, 0.45. Look once again at figure 2. The numbers on the right of the decimal point represent tenths, hundredths, and thousandths, in that order. When you see a decimal fraction, stop, and look closely at the number representing the **tenths**. **The fraction with the highest number representing tenths has the higher value.**

EXAMPLE 1   0.3 is higher than 0.2

EXAMPLE 2   0.41 is higher than 0.29

EXAMPLE 3   1.21 is higher than 1.19

PROBLEM

Which of the following decimals has the highest value?

1. a) 0.3   b) 0.2   c) 0.5

2. a) 2.73   b) 2.61   c) 2.87

3. a) 0.19   b) 0.61   c) 0.34

ANSWERS 1. c 2. c 3. b

If in decimal fractions the numbers representing the tenths are identical, for example, 0.25 and 0.27, then **the number representing the hundredths will determine the relative value**. Once again the **higher** number will have the **higher** value.

EXAMPLE 1   0.27 is higher than 0.25

EXAMPLE 2   0.15 is higher than 0.1 (0.1 is the same as 0.10)

Extra zeros on the end of decimal fractions are omitted because they can cause confusion, although they do not alter the value of the fraction (0.10 is the same as 0.1).

EXAMPLE 3   2.25 is higher than 2.2 (same as 2.20)

EXAMPLE 4   9.77 is higher than 9.75

PROBLEM

Which of the following decimals has the highest value?

1. a) 0.12   b) 0.15   c) 0.17

2. a) 1.21   b) 1.24   c) 1.23

3. a) 0.37   b) 0.32   c) 0.36

ANSWERS 1. c 2. b 3. a

PROBLEM

Which decimal fraction has the higher value?

a) 0.125   b) 0.25

ANSWER   The correct answer is b), 0.25

The decimal fraction which has the higher number representing the **tenths** has the higher value. **2** is higher than **1**; therefore, 0.25 has a higher value than 0.125. Medication errors have been made in this **identical** decimal fraction; so remember it well. **The number of figures on the right of the decimal point is not an indication of relative value. Always look at the figure representing the tenths first, and if these are identical, the hundredths, to determine which is higher.**

This completes your introduction to the relative value of decimals. The rules just reviewed will cover all situations in dosage calculations where you will have to recognize high and low values. Therefore, you are now ready to test yourself on this information.

PROBLEM

Identify the decimal with the highest value in each of the following.

1. a) 0.25   b) 0.5   c) 0.125   _0.5   b_

2. a) 0.4   b) 0.45   c) 0.5   _0.5   c_

3. a) 7.5   b) 6.25   c) 4.75   _7.5   a_

4. a) 0.3   b) 0.25   c) 0.35   _0.35   c_

5. a) 1.125   b) 1.75   c) 1.5   _1.75   b_

6. a) 4.5   b) 4.75   c) 4.25   _4.75   b_

7. a) 0.1   b) 0.01   c) 0.04   _0.1   a_

8. a) 5.75   b) 6.25   c) 6.5   _6.5   c_

9. a) 0.6   b) 0.16   c) 0.06   _0.6   a_

10. a) 3.55   b) 2.95   c) 3.7   _3.7   c_

11. a) 0.015   b) 0.15   c) 0.1   _0.15   b_

12. a) 1.3   b) 1.25   c) 1.35   _1.35   c_

13. a) 0.1   b) 0.2   c) 0.25   _0.25   c_

14. a) 0.125   b) 0.1   c) 0.05   _.125   a_

15. a) 13.7   b) 13.5   c) 13.25   _13.7   a_

ANSWERS 1. b 2. c 3. a 4. c 5. b 6. b 7. a 8. c 9. a 10. c 11. b 12. c 13. c 14. a 15. a

• ADDITION AND SUBTRACTION OF DECIMALS •

There are several basic rules which will make addition and subtraction of decimals safer. Let's look at these.

RULE: When you first write the numbers down, line up decimal points.

EXAMPLE To add 0.25 and 0.27

0.25
0.27 is safe

0.25
0.27 may be unsafe, it could lead to errors.

RULE: Always add or subtract from right to left. If you found it necessary to write the numbers down, don't confuse yourself by trying to "eyeball" the answer. Also, write any numbers carried, or rewrite those reduced by borrowing if you find this helpful.

EXAMPLE 1 When adding 0.25 and 0.27

1
0.25
0.27
─────
0.52

add the 5 and 7 first, then the 2, 2, and the 1 you carried. Right to left.

EXAMPLE 2   When subtracting 0.63 from 0.71

```
   6
0.71
0.63
─────
0.08
```
borrow 1 from the 7 and rewrite as 6, write the borrowed 1. Subtract 3 from 11. Subtract 6 from 6. Work from right to left.

RULE: Add zeros as necessary to make the fractions of equal length. This does not alter the value of the fractions and it helps prevent confusion and mistakes.

EXAMPLE   When subtracting 0.125 from 0.25

```
0.25           0.250
0.125  becomes 0.125      Answer = 0.125
```

If you follow these rules and make them a habit you will automatically reduce calculation errors. The following problems will give you an excellent opportunity to practice them.

PROBLEM

Add the following decimals.

1. 0.25 + 0.5 = .75
2. 0.1 + 2.25 = 2.35
3. 1.7 + 0.75 = 2.45
4. 1.4 + 0.02 = 1.42
5. 2.3 + 1.45 = 3.75

6. 3.7 + 1.05 + 2.2 = 6.95
7. 6.42 + 13.3 + 9.55 = 29.27
8. 5.57 + 4.03 + 13.02 = 22.62
9. 0.33 + 8.41 + 6.09 = 14.83
10. 7.44 + 3.04 + 11.31 = 21.79

Subtract the following decimals.

11. 1.25 − 1.125 = 0.125
12. 3.2 − 0.65 = 2.55
13. 2.3 − 1.45 = 0.85
14. 0.02 − 0.01 = 0.01
15. 5 − 2.5 = 2.5

16. 7.33 − 4.04 = 3.29
17. 12.45 − 2.07 = 10.38
18. 0.07 − 0.035 = 0.035
19. 1.175 − 0.23 = 0.945
20. 5.75 − 0.95 = 4.80

ANSWERS 1. 0.75 **2.** 2.35 **3.** 2.45 **4.** 1.42 **5.** 3.75 **6.** 6.95 **7.** 29.27 **8.** 22.62 **9.** 14.83 **10.** 21.79 **11.** 0.125 **12.** 2.55 **13.** 0.85 **14.** 0.01 **15.** 2.5 **16.** 3.29 **17.** 10.38 **18.** 0.035 **19.** 0.945 **20.** 4.8

This concludes the refresher on relative value, addition, and subtraction of decimals. The important points to remember from this chapter are:

■ a zero is placed in front of a decimal fraction to emphasize the decimal point

■ the number representing the tenths in a decimal fraction is the first determiner of relative value

■ if the tenths in decimal fractions are identical, the number representing hundredths will determine relative value

■ when adding or subtracting decimal fractions, first line up the decimal points then add or subtract from right to left

SUMMARY SELF TEST
Relative Value, Addition, Subtraction of Decimals

DIRECTIONS Choose the decimal with the highest value from each of the following.

1. a) 2.45   b) 2.57   c) 2.19   _b_

2. a) 3.07   b) 3.17   c) 3.71   _c_

3. a) 0.12   b) 0.02   c) 0.01   _a_

4. a) 5.31   b) 5.35   c) 6.01   _c_

5. a) 4.5   b) 4.51   c) 4.15   _b_

6. If you have medication tablets whose strength is 0.1 mg, and you must give 0.3 mg, you will need

    a) 1 tablet   b) less than 1 tablet   c) more than 1 tablet   _c_

7. If you have tablets with a strength of 0.25 mg and you must give 0.125 mg you will need

    a) 1 tablet   b) less than 1 tablet   c) more than 1 tablet   _b_

8. If you have an order to give a dosage of 7.5 mg and the tablets have a strength of 3.75 mg you will need

    a) 1 tablet   b) less than 1 tablet   c) more than 1 tablet   _c_

9. If the order is to give 0.5 mg and the tablet strength is 0.5 mg you will give

    a) 1 tablet   b) less than 1 tablet   c) more than 1 tablet   _a_

10. The order is to give 0.5 mg and the tablets have a strength of 0.25 mg. You must give

    a) 1 tablet   b) less than 1 tablet   c) more than 1 tablet   _c_

DIRECTIONS Add the following decimals.

11. 1.31 + 0.4 = _1.71_   **15.** 1.3 + 1.04 + 0.7 = _3.04_

12. 0.15 + 0.25 = _.40_   **16.** 4.1 + 3.03 + 0.4 = _7.53_

13. 2.5 + 0.75 = _3.25_   **17.** 0.5 + 0.5 + 0.5 = _1.5_

14. 3.2 + 2.17 = _5.37_   **18.** 5.4 + 2.6 + 0.09 = _8.09_

19. You have just given 2 tablets with a dosage strength of 3.5 mg each. What was the total dosage administered? _____7.0 mg_____

20. You are to give your patient one tablet labeled 0.5 mg and one labeled 0.25 mg. What is the total dosage of these two tablets? ___0.75 mg___

21. If you give two tablets labeled 0.02 mg what total dosage will you administer?
_____0.04 mg_____

22. You are to give one tablet labeled 0.8 mg and two tablets labeled 0.4 mg. What is the total dosage? _____1.60 mg_____

23. You have two tablets, one is labeled 0.15 mg and the other 0.3 mg. What is the total dosage of these two tablets? _____0.45 mg_____

DIRECTIONS Subtract the following decimals.

24. $4.32 - 3.1 =$ _____1.22_____   28. $1.3 - 0.02 =$ _____1.28_____
25. $2.1 - 1.91 =$ _____0.19_____   29. $0.2 - 0.07 =$ _____0.13_____
26. $3.7 - 1.93 =$ _____1.77_____   30. $3.95 - 0.35 =$ _____3.60_____
27. $5.75 - 4.02 =$ _____1.73_____   31. $1.9 - 0.08 =$ _____1.82_____

32. Your patient is to receive a dosage of 7.5 mg and you have only one tablet labeled 3.75 mg. How many more milligrams must you give? _____3.75_____

33. You have a tablet labeled 0.02 mg and your patient is to receive 0.06 mg. How many more milligrams do you need? _____.04_____

34. The tablet available is labeled 0.5 mg but you must give a dosage of 1.5 mg. How many more milligrams will you need to obtain the correct dosage?
_____1.0_____

35. Your patient is to receive a dosage of 1.2 mg and you have one tablet labeled 0.6 mg. What additional dosage in milligrams will you need? _____.60_____

36. You must give your patient a dosage of 2.2 mg but have only two tablets labeled 0.55 mg. What additional dosage in milligrams will you need?
_____1.1_____

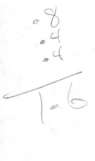

2
Multiplication and Division of Decimals

OBJECTIVES
The student will
1. define product, numerator and denominator
2. multiply decimal fractions
3. reduce fractions using common denominators
4. divide fractions and express answers to the nearest tenth, and hundredth

INTRODUCTION
Multiplication and division of decimals is a routine part of calculating drug dosages. This is an area where using a calculator may be helpful. For the purpose of understanding and review, however, you may wish to do the following exercises without one. Let's begin with multiplication.

• MULTIPLICATION OF DECIMALS •

The main precaution in multiplication of decimals is the **placement of the decimal point in the answer** (which is called the **product**).

> **RULE: The decimal point in the product of decimal fractions is placed the same number of places to the left as the total of numbers after the decimal point in the fractions multiplied.**

EXAMPLE 1 0.35×0.5

Begin by lining the numbers up on the right, since this is somewhat safer; and disregard the decimals during the actual multiplication.

$$
\begin{array}{r}
0.35 \\
\underline{0.5} \\
175
\end{array} \qquad \text{Answer} = 0.175
$$

0.35 has two numbers after the decimal, 0.5 has one. Place the decimal point three places to the left in the product. Place a zero (0) in front of the decimal to emphasize it.

EXAMPLE 2
$$
\begin{array}{r}
1.4 \\
\underline{0.25} \\
70 \\
\underline{28} \\
350
\end{array} \qquad \text{Answer} = 0.35
$$

1.4 has one number after the decimal, 0.25 has two. Place the decimal point three places to the left in the product, and add a zero in front (0.350). Once the decimal is correctly placed the excess zero is dropped from the end of the fraction, and 0.350 becomes 0.35

RULE: If the product contains insufficient numbers for correct placement of the decimal point, add as many zeros as necessary to the left of the product to correct this.

EXAMPLE 3   0.21
　　　　　　　　　0.32
　　　　　　　　　─────
　　　　　　　　　42
　　　　　　　　　63
　　　　　　　　　─────
　　　　　　　　　672　　　　　Answer = 0.0672

In this example 0.21 has two numbers after the decimal, and 0.32 also has two. However, there are only three numbers in the product, so a zero must be added to the left of these numbers to place the decimal point correctly: 672 becomes 0.0672

EXAMPLE 4   0.12
　　　　　　　　　0.2
　　　　　　　　　─────
　　　　　　　　　24　　　　　Answer = 0.024

There are a total of three numbers after the decimal points in 0.12 and 0.2. One zero must be added in the product to place the decimal point correctly: 24 becomes 0.024

PROBLEM

Multiply the following decimal fractions.

1. 0.45 × 0.2 = _____ .09
2. 1.3 × 0.15 = _____ .0195
3. 3.5 × 1.2 = _____ 4.20
4. 2.2 × 1.1 = _____ 2.42
5. 1.3 × 0.05 = _____ .065
6. 6.25 × 3.2 = _____ 20.

7. 0.7 × 0.05 = _____ .035
8. 12.5 × 2.2 = _____ 27.50
9. 16 × 0.3 = _____ 4.4
10. 0.4 × 0.17 = _____ 0.08
11. 2.14 × 0.9 = _____ 1.926
12. 0.35 × 1.9 = _____ .665

ANSWERS 1. 0.09 2. 0.195 3. 4.2 4. 2.42 5. 0.065 6. 20 7. 0.035 8. 27.5 9. 4.8 10. 0.068
11. 1.926 12. 0.665

• DIVISION OF DECIMALS •

Look at this sample division:

$$\frac{0.25}{0.125} = \frac{numerator}{denominator}$$

You may recall that the **top number**, 0.25, is called the **numerator** while the **bottom number**, 0.125, is called the **denominator**. (If you have trouble remembering which is which, think of D, for down, for denominator, the denominator is on the bottom). With this basic terminology reviewed we are now ready to look at two preliminary math steps which are used to simplify the fraction prior to final division. The first step is to eliminate the decimal points completely.

• ELIMINATION OF DECIMAL POINTS •

Decimal points can be eliminated from the numbers in a decimal fraction without changing its value.

> **RULE: To eliminate the decimal points from decimal fractions move them the same number of places to the right in both the numerator and the denominator until they are eliminated in both. Zeros may have to be added to accomplish this.**

EXAMPLE 1 $\dfrac{0.25}{0.125}$ becomes $\dfrac{250}{125}$

The decimal point must be moved three places to the right in 0.125 to make it 125. Therefore it must be moved three places in 0.25, which requires the addition of one zero to make it 250.

EXAMPLE 2 $\dfrac{0.3}{0.15}$ becomes $\dfrac{30}{15}$

The decimal point must be moved two places in 0.15 to make it 15. It must be moved two places in 0.3, which requires the addition of one zero to become 30.

EXAMPLE 3 $\dfrac{1.5}{2}$ becomes $\dfrac{15}{20}$

Move the decimal point one place in 1.5 to make it 15; add one zero to 2 to make it 20.

EXAMPLE 4 $\dfrac{4.5}{0.95}$ becomes $\dfrac{450}{95}$

Remember that moving the decimal point does not alter the value of the fraction or the answer you will obtain in the final division. It just makes the numbers easier to work with. Now try some problems on your own.

PROBLEM

Eliminate the decimal points from the following decimal fractions.

1. $\dfrac{17.5}{2}$ = _____

2. $\dfrac{0.5}{25}$ = _____

3. $\dfrac{6.3}{0.6}$ = _____

4. $\dfrac{3.76}{0.4}$ = _____

5. $\dfrac{8.4}{0.7}$ = _____

6. $\dfrac{0.1}{0.05}$ = _____

7. $\dfrac{0.9}{0.03} =$ _____   *90/3*   9. $\dfrac{0.4}{0.04} =$ _____ *40/4*

8. $\dfrac{10.75}{2.5} =$ _____ *1075/25*   10. $\dfrac{1.2}{0.4} =$ _____ *12/4*

ANSWERS 1. $\dfrac{175}{20}$ 2. $\dfrac{5}{250}$ 3. $\dfrac{63}{6}$ 4. $\dfrac{376}{40}$ 5. $\dfrac{84}{7}$ 6. $\dfrac{10}{5}$ 7. $\dfrac{90}{3}$ 8. $\dfrac{1075}{250}$ 9. $\dfrac{40}{4}$ 10. $\dfrac{12}{4}$

• REDUCTION OF FRACTIONS •

Once the decimal points are eliminated the next step is to reduce the numbers as far as possible.

RULE: To reduce fractions divide both numbers by their highest common denominator (the highest number which will divide into both). This is usually 2, 3, 4, 5, or multiples of these numbers, such as 6, 8, 25, and so on.

EXAMPLE 1 $\dfrac{175}{20}$ The highest common denominator is 5

$$\dfrac{175}{20} = \dfrac{35}{4}$$

EXAMPLE 2 $\dfrac{63}{6}$ The highest common denominator is 3

$$\dfrac{63}{6} = \dfrac{21}{2}$$

EXAMPLE 3 $\dfrac{1075}{250}$ The highest common denominator is 25

$$\dfrac{1075}{250} = \dfrac{43}{10}$$

There is a second way you could have reduced the fraction in example 3, and it is equally as correct. Divide by 5, then 5 again.

$$\dfrac{1075}{250} = \dfrac{215}{50} = \dfrac{43}{10}$$

RULE: If the highest common denominator is difficult to determine, reduce several times by using lower common denominators.

EXAMPLE 4 $\dfrac{376}{40} = \dfrac{47}{5}$ Reduce by 8 or divide by 4, then 2 $\dfrac{\cancel{376}}{\cancel{40}} = \dfrac{\cancel{94}}{\cancel{10}} = \dfrac{47}{5}$

or divide by 2, 2, and 2 $\dfrac{\cancel{376}}{\cancel{40}} = \dfrac{\cancel{188}}{\cancel{20}} = \dfrac{\cancel{94}}{\cancel{10}} = \dfrac{47}{5}$

Remember that simple numbers are easiest to work with, and the time spent in extra reductions may be well worth the payoff in safety.

PROBLEM

Reduce the following fractions as much as possible in preparation for final division.

1. $\dfrac{84}{8} =$ $\dfrac{42}{4} = \dfrac{21}{2}$

2. $\dfrac{20}{16} =$ $\dfrac{5}{4}$

3. $\dfrac{250}{325} =$ $\dfrac{10}{13}$

4. $\dfrac{96}{34} =$ $\dfrac{48}{17}$

5. $\dfrac{175}{20} =$ $\dfrac{35}{4}$

6. $\dfrac{40}{14} =$ $\dfrac{20}{7}$

7. $\dfrac{84}{28} =$ $\dfrac{21}{7}$

8. $\dfrac{100}{75} =$ $\dfrac{4}{3}$

9. $\dfrac{50}{75} =$ $\dfrac{2}{3}$

10. $\dfrac{60}{88} =$ $\dfrac{30}{44} = \dfrac{15}{22}$

ANSWERS   1. $\dfrac{21}{2}$ 2. $\dfrac{5}{4}$ 3. $\dfrac{10}{13}$ 4. $\dfrac{48}{17}$ 5. $\dfrac{35}{4}$ 6. $\dfrac{20}{7}$ 7. $\dfrac{21}{7}$ 8. $\dfrac{4}{3}$ 9. $\dfrac{2}{3}$ 10. $\dfrac{15}{22}$

• REDUCTION OF NUMBERS ENDING IN ZERO •

There is one other type of reduction which, while not directly related to decimal fractions, is best covered at this time. This concerns reductions when both numbers in the fraction end with zeros.

EXAMPLE $\dfrac{2500}{500}$

RULE: Fractions in which both the numerator and denominator end in a zero or zeros, may be reduced by crossing off the same number of zeros in each.

EXAMPLE 1 $\dfrac{800}{250}$

In this fraction the numerator, 800, has two zeros, and the denominator, 250, has one zero. The number of zeros crossed off must be the same in both numerator and denominator, so only one zero can be eliminated from each.

$\dfrac{80\cancel{0}}{25\cancel{0}} = \dfrac{80}{25}$

EXAMPLE 2 $\dfrac{24\cancel{00}}{20\cancel{00}} = \dfrac{24}{20}$

Two zeros can be eliminated from the denominator and numerator in this fraction.

EXAMPLE 3 $\dfrac{15\cancel{000}}{30\cancel{000}} = \dfrac{15}{30}$

In this fraction three zeros can be eliminated.

PROBLEM

Reduce the following fractions in preparation for final division.

1. $\dfrac{50}{250}$ = _____ $\dfrac{5}{25} = \dfrac{1}{5}$ _____

6. $\dfrac{110}{100}$ = _____ $\dfrac{11}{10}$ _____

2. $\dfrac{120}{50}$ = _____ $\dfrac{12}{5}$ _____

7. $\dfrac{200{,}000}{150{,}000}$ = _____ $\dfrac{20}{15} = \dfrac{4}{3}$ _____

3. $\dfrac{2500}{1500}$ = _____ $\dfrac{25}{15} = \dfrac{5}{3}$ _____

8. $\dfrac{1000}{800}$ = _____ $\dfrac{10}{8} = \dfrac{5}{4}$ _____

4. $\dfrac{1{,}000{,}000}{750{,}000}$ = _____ $\dfrac{100}{75} = \dfrac{4}{3}$ _____

9. $\dfrac{60}{40}$ = _____ $\dfrac{6}{4} = \dfrac{3}{2}$ _____

5. $\dfrac{800}{150}$ = _____ $\dfrac{80}{15} = \dfrac{16}{3}$ _____

10. $\dfrac{150}{200}$ = _____ $\dfrac{15}{20} = \dfrac{3}{4}$ _____

ANSWERS   1. $\dfrac{1}{5}$ 2. $\dfrac{12}{5}$ 3. $\dfrac{5}{3}$ 4. $\dfrac{4}{3}$ 5. $\dfrac{16}{3}$ 6. $\dfrac{11}{10}$ 7. $\dfrac{4}{3}$ 8. $\dfrac{5}{4}$ 9. $\dfrac{3}{2}$ 10. $\dfrac{3}{4}$

• EXPRESSING TO THE NEAREST TENTH •

When a fraction is reduced as much as possible it is ready for final division. Answers are most often rounded off and expressed as decimal numbers to the nearest tenth.

RULE: To express an answer to the nearest tenth the division is carried to hundredths. When the number representing hundredths is 5 or larger, the number representing tenths is increased by one.

EXAMPLE 1 $\dfrac{35}{4}$ =   8.75

Answer   =   8.8

The number representing hundredths is 5, so the number representing tenths is increased by one. 8.7 becomes 8.8

EXAMPLE 2   5.19 is expressed as 5.2

The number representing hundredths, 9, is larger then 5, and 1 becomes 2

EXAMPLE 3   0.97 becomes 1

The number representing hundreths is 7, so 9 becomes 1.0 which is expressed as 1

EXAMPLE 4   2.43 remains 2.4

The number representing hundredths, 3, is less than 5, so the number representing tenths, 4, does not change.

EXAMPLE 5   1.42 remains 1.4

EXAMPLE 6   1.86 becomes 1.9

PROBLEM

Express the following numbers to the nearest tenth.

1. 3.27 = _3.3_   7. 0.96 = _1.0_
2. 3.51 = _3.5_   8. 2.15 = _2.1_
3. 2.92 = _2.9_   9. 1.18 = _1.2_
4. 1.99 = _2.0_   10. 2.73 = _2.7_
5. 0.74 = _.7_   11. 3.09 = _3.1_
6. 1.03 = _1.0_   12. 0.41 = _.4_

ANSWERS   **1.** 3.3   **2.** 3.5   **3.** 2.9   **4.** 2   **5.** 0.7   **6.** 1   **7.** 1   **8.** 2.2   **9.** 1.2   **10.** 2.7   **11.** 3.1   **12.** 0.4

• EXPRESSING TO THE NEAREST HUNDREDTH •

Some drugs are administered in dosages carried to the nearest hundredth.

RULE: To express an answer to the nearest hundredth the division is carried to thousandths. When the number representing thousandths is 5 or larger, the number representing hundredths is increased by one. Carry the division to three places after the decimal point to determine thousandths.

EXAMPLE 1   0.736 becomes 0.74

The number representing thousandths, 6, is larger than 5, so the number representing hundredths, 3, is increased by 1 to become 4.

EXAMPLE 2   0.777 becomes 0.78

EXAMPLE 3   0.373 remains 0.37

The number representing thousandths, 3, is less than five, so the number representing hundredths, 7, remains unchanged.

EXAMPLE 4   0.934 remains 0.93

PROBLEM

Express the following numbers to the nearest hundredth.

1. 0.175 = _____0.18_____   7. 1.081 = _____1.08_____
2. 0.344 = _____0.34_____   8. 1.327 = _____1.33_____
3. 1.853 = _____1.85_____   9. 0.739 = _____0.74_____
4. 0.306 = _____.31_____   10. 0.733 = _____0.73_____
5. 3.015 = _____3.02_____   11. 2.072 = _____2.07_____
6. 2.154 = _____2.15_____   12. 0.089 = _____0.09_____

ANSWERS **1.** 0.18 **2.** 0.34 **3.** 1.85 **4.** 0.31 **5.** 3.02 **6.** 2.15 **7.** 1.08 **8.** 1.33 **9.** 0.74 **10.** 0.73
11. 2.07 **12.** 0.09

This concludes the chapter on multiplication and division of decimals. The important points to remember from this chapter are:

■ when decimal fractions are multiplied the decimal point is placed the same number of places to the left in the product as the total of numbers after the decimal points in the fractions multiplied

■ zeros must be placed in front of a product if it contains insufficient numbers for correct placement of the decimal point

■ to simplify division of decimal fractions the preliminary steps of eliminating the decimal points, and reducing the numbers by common denominators can be used

■ when fractions are divided answers are expressed as decimal fractions to the nearest tenth, or the nearest hundredth

SUMMARY SELF TEST
Multiplication and Division of Decimals

DIRECTIONS   Multiply the following decimals.

1. 1.49×0.05 = _____.0745_____   6. 5.3×1.02 = _____5.406_____
2. 0.15×3.04 = _____.4560_____   7. 0.35×1.25 = _____.4375_____
3. 0.025×3.5 = _____.0875_____   8. 4.32×0.05 = _____.2160_____
4. 0.55×2.5 = _____1.375_____   9. 0.2×0.02 = _____.004_____
5. 1.31×2.07 = _____2.7117_____   10. 0.4×1.75 = _____.700_____

11. You are to administer four tablets with a dosage strength of 0.04 mg each, what total dosage are you giving? _____.16_____

12. You have given 2½ (2.5) tablets with a strength of 1.25 mg, what total dosage is this? _____3.125_____   or 3.13 rounded

13. The tablets your patient is to receive are labeled 0.1 mg and you are to give 3½ (3.5) tablets. What total dosage is this? _____.35_____

14. You gave your patient 3 tablets labeled 0.75 mg each, and he was to receive a total of 2.25 mg; did he receive the correct dosage? _____Yes_____

15. The tablets available for your patient are labeled 12.5 mg, and you are to give 4½ (4.5) tablets. What total dosage will this be? _____52.25_____

16. Your patient is to receive a dosage of 4.5 mg. The tablets available are labeled 3.5 mg, and there are 2½ tablets in his medication drawer. Is this a correct dosage? _____No_____   8.75

DIRECTIONS Divide the following fractions and express your answers to the nearest tenth.

17. $\dfrac{1.3}{0.7}$ = _____1.9_____

18. $\dfrac{1.9}{3.2}$ = _____.6_____

19. $\dfrac{32.5}{9}$ = _____3.6_____

20. $\dfrac{0.04}{0.1}$ = _____.4_____

21. $\dfrac{1.45}{1.2}$ = _____1.2_____

22. $\dfrac{250}{1000}$ = _____.3_____

23. $\dfrac{0.8}{0.09}$ = _____8.9_____

24. $\dfrac{2,000,000}{1,500,000}$ = _____1.3_____

25. $\dfrac{4.1}{2.05}$ = _____2.0_____

26. $\dfrac{7.3}{12}$ = _____.6_____

27. $\dfrac{150,000}{120,000}$ = _____1.3_____

28. $\dfrac{0.15}{0.08}$ = _____1.9_____

29. $\dfrac{2700}{900}$ = _____3.0_____

30. $\dfrac{0.25}{0.15}$ = _____1.7_____

$0.7 \overline{)1.3^{4}00}$

DIRECTIONS Divide the following fractions and express your answers to the nearest hundredth.

31. $\dfrac{2000}{1700}$ = _____1.18_____

32. $\dfrac{0.125}{0.3}$ = _____.42_____

33. $\dfrac{1450}{1500}$ = _____ .97_____

34. $\dfrac{325}{175}$ = _____ 1.86_____

35. $\dfrac{0.6}{1.35}$ = _____ .44_____

36. $\dfrac{0.04}{0.12}$ = _____ .33_____

37. $\dfrac{750}{10,000}$ = _____ .06_____

38. $\dfrac{0.65}{0.8}$ = _____ .81_____

39. $\dfrac{3.01}{4.2}$ = _____ .72_____

40. $\dfrac{4.5}{6.1}$ = _____ .74_____

ANSWERS

1. 0.0745   **2.** 0.456   **3.** 0.0875   **4.** 1.375   **5.** 2.7117   **6.** 5.406   **7.** 0.4375   **8.** 0.216   **9.** 0.004   **10.** 0.7   **11.** 0.16 mg
12. 3.125 mg   **13.** 0.35 mg   **14.** Yes   **15.** 56.25 mg   **16.** No   **17.** 1.9   **18.** 0.6   **19.** 3.6   **20.** 0.4   **21.** 1.2   **22.** 0.3   **23.** 8.9
24. 1.3   **25.** 2   **26.** 0.6   **27.** 1.3   **28.** 1.9   **29.** 3   **30.** 1.7   **31.** 1.18   **32.** 0.42   **33.** 0.97   **34.** 1.86   **35.** 0.44   **36.** 0.33
37. 0.08   **38.** 0.81   **39.** 0.72   **40.** 0.74

3
Math of Common Fractions

OBJECTIVES
The student will
1. identify which of several common fractions has the highest (or lowest) value
2. multiply common fractions
3. divide common fractions

INTRODUCTION
The math involving common fractions covered in this chapter is necessary because you may encounter calculations requiring the use of the apothecaries' system, which uses common fractions. This review will cover three essentials: relative value, multiplication, and division. We will start with a review of relative value, so that you will be able to recognize which fractions have the highest (and lowest) value.

• RELATIVE VALUE OF COMMON FRACTIONS •

Let's start this review by looking at the common fractions $\frac{1}{2}$ and $\frac{1}{4}$. The numerator in

both fractions is 1; 2 and 4 are the denominators.

> **RULE: When the numerators are the same the fraction with the lowest denominator has the highest value.** 2 is a lower number than 4, so

$\frac{1}{2}$ has a higher value than $\frac{1}{4}$

Here is a memory cue to help you remember this rule. Think of an aspirin tablet: $\frac{1}{2}$ an

aspirin is larger than $\frac{1}{4}$ of an aspirin. The lower denominator, 2, has the higher value.

Figure 3 graphically illustrates this.

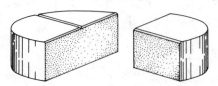

Figure 3

EXAMPLE 1 $\frac{1}{3}$ is higher than $\frac{1}{8}$ because 3 is a lower denominator than 8

EXAMPLE 2 $\dfrac{1}{100}$ is higher than $\dfrac{1}{150}$

EXAMPLE 3 $\dfrac{1}{150}$ is higher than $\dfrac{1}{200}$

RULE: If the denominators are the same, the fraction with the higher numerator will have the higher value.

EXAMPLE 1 $\dfrac{3}{10}$ is higher than $\dfrac{1}{10}$

The denominators, 10, are the same, so the numerator 3, gives the first fraction the highest value.

EXAMPLE 2 $\dfrac{4}{5}$ is higher than $\dfrac{2}{5}$

In drug dosages the numerator is almost always 1, so the relative value is determined by the denominator, for example $\dfrac{1}{4}, \dfrac{1}{100}$

PROBLEM

Identify the fraction with the highest value in each of the following.

1. a) $\dfrac{1}{3}$ b) $\dfrac{1}{6}$ c) $\dfrac{1}{4}$ _a_____

2. a) $\dfrac{1}{8}$ b) $\dfrac{1}{6}$ c) $\dfrac{1}{4}$ _c_____

3. a) $\dfrac{1}{4}$ b) $\dfrac{1}{8}$ c) $\dfrac{1}{5}$ _a_____

4. a) $\dfrac{1}{75}$ b) $\dfrac{1}{50}$ c) $\dfrac{1}{100}$ _b_____

5. a) $\dfrac{1}{2}$ b) $\dfrac{1}{6}$ c) $\dfrac{1}{4}$ _a_____

6. a) $\dfrac{1}{200}$ b) $\dfrac{1}{150}$ c) $\dfrac{1}{100}$ _c_____

7. a) $\dfrac{3}{32}$ b) $\dfrac{4}{32}$ c) $\dfrac{1}{32}$ _b_____

8. a) $\dfrac{1}{10}$ b) $\dfrac{1}{15}$ c) $\dfrac{1}{5}$ _c_____

9. a) $\dfrac{1}{5}$ b) $\dfrac{3}{5}$ c) $\dfrac{2}{5}$ _____ b

10. a) $\dfrac{1}{3}$ b) $\dfrac{1}{2}$ c) $\dfrac{1}{4}$ _____ b

ANSWERS   1. a   2. c   3. a   4. b   5. a   6. c   7. b   8. c   9. b   10. b

• MULTIPLICATION OF COMMON FRACTIONS •

Multiplication of common fractions will include **proper fractions** in which the **numerator is smaller than the denominator**, for example $\dfrac{1}{4}$; and **improper fractions**, in which the **numerator is larger than the denominator**, for example $\dfrac{5}{4}$

Regardless of the type of fraction, multiplication of common fractions in dosage calculations has three steps: reduction of the numbers (if this is possible); multiplication of the remaining numerators, then the remaining denominators; and finally, division of the remaining fraction to express the answer as a decimal number, usually to the nearest tenth. Let's look at some examples.

EXAMPLE 1 $\dfrac{1}{6} \times \dfrac{2}{3}$

$\dfrac{1}{6_3} \times \dfrac{2^1}{3}$ reduce the fractions

$\dfrac{1}{9}$ multiply the remaining numerators ($1 \times 1 = 1$)
then the denominators ($3 \times 3 = 9$)

$1 \div 9$ divide the final fraction to two places after the decimal point

0.1   express as a decimal fraction to the nearest tenth

EXAMPLE 2 $\dfrac{7}{50} \times \dfrac{25}{3}$

$\dfrac{7}{50_2} \times \dfrac{25^1}{3}$ reduce; multiply numerators, then denominators

$\dfrac{7}{6}$ divide remaining fraction

$1.16 = \textbf{1.2}$ express answer to nearest tenth

As you can see this math is uncomplicated, and you are now ready for some problems on your own.

PROBLEM

Multiply the following common fractions. Express answers as decimal numbers to the nearest tenth.

1. $\dfrac{1}{8} \times \dfrac{6}{1} =$ ___.8___   6. $\dfrac{2}{9} \times \dfrac{3}{5} =$ ___.1___

2. $\dfrac{3}{5} \times \dfrac{10}{5} =$ ___1.2___   7. $\dfrac{1}{6} \times \dfrac{10}{1} =$ ___1.7___

3. $\dfrac{2}{7} \times \dfrac{8}{4} =$ ___.6___   8. $\dfrac{7}{12} \times \dfrac{4}{10} =$ ___.2___

4. $\dfrac{1}{50} \times \dfrac{100}{1} =$ ___2___   9. $\dfrac{7}{8} \times \dfrac{2}{21} =$ ___.1___

5. $\dfrac{1}{3} \times \dfrac{4}{1} =$ ___1.3___   10. $\dfrac{1}{5} \times \dfrac{3}{1} =$ ___.6___

ANSWERS   **1.** 0.8   **2.** 1.2   **3.** 0.6   **4.** 2   **5.** 1.3   **6.** 0.1   **7.** 1.7   **8.** 0.2   **9.** 0.1   **10.** 0.6

• DIVISION OF COMMON FRACTIONS •

When a dosage calculation involves the division of one common fraction by another it will be written as follows:

$$\dfrac{\dfrac{1}{3}}{\dfrac{1}{6}} \qquad \dfrac{1}{3} \text{ is a numerator, } \dfrac{1}{6} \text{ is a denominator}$$

RULE: To divide common fractions the fraction representing the denominator is inverted (turned upside down), and the problem is converted to an equivalent multiplication.

EXAMPLE 1

$$\dfrac{\dfrac{1}{3}}{\dfrac{1}{6}} \quad \text{becomes} \quad \dfrac{1}{3} \times \dfrac{6}{1}$$

The denominator, $\dfrac{1}{6}$, is inverted to become $\dfrac{6}{1}$, and the problem is converted to a multiplication.

$$\dfrac{1}{\cancel{3}_1} \times \dfrac{\cancel{6}^2}{1} = \dfrac{2}{1} = \mathbf{2}$$

EXAMPLE 2

$$\frac{\dfrac{1}{150}}{\dfrac{1}{100}} \quad \text{becomes} \quad \frac{1}{150} \times \frac{100}{1}$$

$$\frac{1}{\cancel{150}_3} \times \frac{\cancel{100}^2}{1}$$

$$\frac{2}{3} = 0.66 = \mathbf{0.7}$$

EXAMPLE 3

$$\frac{\dfrac{1}{10}}{\dfrac{1}{8}} \quad \text{becomes} \quad \frac{1}{10} \times \frac{8}{1}$$

$$\frac{1}{\cancel{10}_5} \times \frac{\cancel{8}^4}{1}$$

$$\frac{4}{5} = \mathbf{0.8}$$

PROBLEM

Divide the following common fractions. Express your answers as decimal numbers to the nearest tenth.

1. $$\frac{\dfrac{1}{50}}{\dfrac{1}{60}} = \underline{\quad 1.2 \quad}$$

2. $$\frac{\dfrac{1}{12}}{\dfrac{1}{4}} = \underline{\quad .3 \quad}$$

3. $$\frac{\dfrac{1}{4}}{\dfrac{1}{6}} = \underline{\quad 1.5 \quad}$$

4. $$\frac{\dfrac{1}{8}}{\dfrac{1}{4}} = \underline{\quad .5 \quad}$$

5. $$\frac{\dfrac{3}{4}}{\dfrac{1}{2}} = \underline{\quad 1.5 \quad}$$

6. $$\frac{\frac{1}{75}}{\frac{1}{150}} = \underline{\qquad 2 \qquad}$$

7. $$\frac{\frac{3}{4}}{\frac{2}{3}} = \underline{\qquad 1.1 \qquad}$$

8. $$\frac{\frac{1}{10}}{\frac{1}{6}} = \underline{\qquad .6 \qquad}$$

9. $$\frac{\frac{1}{100}}{\frac{1}{50}} = \underline{\qquad .5 \qquad}$$

10. $$\frac{\frac{1}{150}}{\frac{1}{200}} = \underline{\qquad 1.3 \qquad}$$

ANSWERS   **1.** 1.2   **2.** 0.3   **3.** 1.5   **4.** 0.5   **5.** 1.5   **6.** 2   **7.** 1.1   **8.** 0.6   **9.** 0.5   **10.** 1.3

This completes your review of the math of common fractions. The important points to remember from this chapter are:

- when the numerators are the same in common fractions the denominator determines relative value

- the lower the denominator the higher the value

- fractions are divided by inverting the fraction representing the denominator, thus converting the problem to an equivalent multiplication

- answers to division and multiplication are expressed as decimal numbers usually to the nearest tenth

SUMMARY SELF TEST

Math of Common Fractions

DIRECTIONS   Identify the fraction with the highest value in each of the following.

1. a) $\frac{1}{60}$ b) $\frac{1}{50}$ c) $\frac{1}{70}$ $\underline{\qquad b \qquad}$

2. a) $\frac{1}{12}$ b) $\frac{1}{10}$ c) $\frac{1}{8}$ $\underline{\qquad c \qquad}$

3. a) $\dfrac{1}{10}$ b) $\dfrac{4}{10}$ c) $\dfrac{9}{10}$ _____ c _____

4. a) $\dfrac{1}{120}$ b) $\dfrac{1}{150}$ c) $\dfrac{1}{175}$ _____ a _____

5. a) $\dfrac{1}{4}$ b) $\dfrac{1}{2}$ c) $\dfrac{1}{3}$ _____ a _____

6. If you had some tablets whose strength was ⅙ and you had to give ¼, you would need

a) less than one tablet   b) more than one tablet _____ b _____

7. If you had some tablets whose strength was ⅟₁₀₀, and you needed to give ⅟₁₅₀, you would need

a) less than one tablet   b) more than one tablet _____ a _____

8. If the tablets available had a strength of ⅕ and you had to give ¼ you would need

a) less than one tablet   b) more than one tablet _____ b _____

9. The order is to give ⅟₁₀ and the tablets available have a strength of ⅛. You will need

a) less than one tablet   b) more than one tablet _____ a _____

10. You have some tablets labeled ⅟₁₀₀ and you must give ⅟₂₀₀. You will need

a) less than one tablet   b) more than one tablet _____ a _____

DIRECTIONS Convert the following divisions to multiplications and express your answers as decimal fractions to the nearest tenth.

11. $\dfrac{\dfrac{1}{2}}{\dfrac{1}{3}} =$ _____ 1.5 _____

12. $\dfrac{\dfrac{1}{4}}{\dfrac{1}{2}} =$ _____ .5 _____

13. $\dfrac{\dfrac{1}{4}}{\dfrac{1}{8}} =$ _____ 2 _____

14. $\dfrac{\dfrac{1}{50}}{\dfrac{1}{75}}$ = _____ 1.5 _____

15. $\dfrac{\dfrac{1}{100}}{\dfrac{1}{150}}$ = _____ 1.5 _____

16. $\dfrac{\dfrac{1}{10}}{\dfrac{1}{12}}$ = _____ 1.2 _____

17. $\dfrac{\dfrac{1}{200}}{\dfrac{1}{150}}$ = _____ .8 _____

18. $\dfrac{\dfrac{1}{3}}{\dfrac{3}{4}}$ = _____ .4 _____

19. $\dfrac{\dfrac{3}{4}}{\dfrac{1}{4}}$ = _____ 3 _____

20. $\dfrac{\dfrac{1}{8}}{\dfrac{5}{6}}$ = _____ .2 _____

21. $\dfrac{\dfrac{1}{8}}{\dfrac{1}{2}}$ = _____ .3 _____

22. $\dfrac{\dfrac{1}{3}}{\dfrac{1}{2}}$ = _____ .7 _____

23.
$$\frac{\frac{2}{3}}{\frac{1}{4}} =$$ _2.7_

24.
$$\frac{\frac{1}{2}}{\frac{1}{6}} =$$ _3_

25.
$$\frac{\frac{1}{6}}{\frac{1}{4}} =$$ _0.7_

26.
$$\frac{\frac{1}{100}}{\frac{1}{200}} =$$ _2_

27.
$$\frac{\frac{1}{300}}{\frac{1}{250}} =$$ _0.8_

28.
$$\frac{\frac{1}{6}}{\frac{1}{5}} =$$ _0.8_

29.
$$\frac{\frac{1}{4}}{\frac{2}{3}} =$$ _0.4_

30.
$$\frac{\frac{1}{80}}{\frac{1}{75}} =$$ _0.9_

ANSWERS

1. b   2. c   3. c   4. a   5. b   6. b   7. a   8. b   9. a   10. a   11. 1.5   12. 0.5   13. 2   14. 1.5   15. 1.5   16. 1.2   17. 0.8
18. 0.4   19. 3   20. 0.2   21. 0.3   22. 0.7   23. 2.7   24. 3   25. 0.7   26. 2   27. 0.8   28. 0.8   29. 0.4   30. 0.9

4

Solving Equations to Determine the Value of X

OBJECTIVES

The student will determine the value of X in
1. equations containing whole numbers
2. equations containing decimal numbers
3. equations containing common fractions

INTRODUCTION

All the clinical calculations you will be doing will ultimately require that you solve an equation to determine the value of an unknown, represented by X. In the previous three chapters you have reviewed all the basic math you will need to do this. In this chapter we will review step-by-step how these math skills are used together to solve for X. Calculations will involve equations containing whole numbers, decimal numbers, and common fractions, and we will review each of these separately.

• WHOLE NUMBER EQUATIONS •

The best way to review this material is by actually working with the equations. Follow each step carefully in the following examples.

EXAMPLE 1 $\dfrac{75}{50} \times 3 = X$

The only reminder you may need to get started is that 3 is a numerator. If you wish you can write it as $\dfrac{3}{1}$

$$\dfrac{75}{50} \times \dfrac{3}{1} = X$$

$\dfrac{\cancel{75}^{3}}{\cancel{50}_{2}} \times \dfrac{3}{1}$ reduce 75 and 50 by their highest common denominator, 25

$\dfrac{3 \times 3}{2 \times 1}$ multiply the remaining numerators, $3 \times 3 = 9$; then the remaining denominators, $2 \times 1 = 2$

$\dfrac{9}{2}$ divide the numerator 9 by the denominator 2

$X = 4.5$ express your answer as a decimal number to the nearest tenth.

EXAMPLE 2 $\dfrac{75,000}{300,000} \times 2 = X$

$\dfrac{75,\cancel{000}}{300,\cancel{000}} \times 2$ reduce the zeros by the same number in one numerator and one denominator.

$\dfrac{\cancel{75}^{1}}{\cancel{300}_{4}} \times 2$ reduce 75 and 300 by 75

$\dfrac{1 \times \cancel{2}^{1}}{\cancel{4}_{2}}$ reduce again by 2

$\dfrac{1}{2}$ divide the final fraction

$X = \mathbf{0.5}$ express the answer as a decimal fraction to the nearest tenth.

EXAMPLE 3 $\dfrac{375}{450} \times 2.5 = X$

It is not uncommon in dosage problems for the second numerator to be a decimal number, as in this equation (2.5). This numerator is usually a small number, and is most easily handled mathematically by keeping it a decimal.

$\dfrac{\cancel{375}^{15}}{\cancel{450}_{18}} \times 2.5 = X$ reduce by 25

$\dfrac{15 \times 2.5}{18}$ multiply the remaining numerators (15 × 2.5)

$\dfrac{37.5}{18}$ divide the final fraction

$X = 2.08 = \mathbf{2.1}$

EXAMPLE 4 $\dfrac{120}{80} \times 1 = X$

In this example the second numerator is 1. In many dosage problems this is the case, and the math to determine the value of X becomes even simpler.

$\dfrac{120}{80} \times 1 = X$ drop the 1 as it has no effect on the equation

$\dfrac{12\cancel{0}}{8\cancel{0}}$ reduce by one zero in the numerator and denominator

$$\frac{\cancel{12}^3}{\cancel{8}_2}$$

reduce again by 4

X = **1.5**

divide the final fraction and express as a decimal number

PROBLEM

Determine the value of X in the following equations. Express your answers to the nearest tenth.

1. $\dfrac{350}{400} \times 3 = X = \underline{\hspace{1em} 2.6 \hspace{1em}}$

2. $\dfrac{175}{100} \times 1 = X = \underline{\hspace{1em} 1.9 \hspace{1em}}$

3. $\dfrac{32}{48} \times 1.4 = X = \underline{\hspace{1em} .9 \hspace{1em}}$

4. $\dfrac{1000}{1250} \times 2.2 = X = \underline{\hspace{1em} 1.8 \hspace{1em}}$

5. $\dfrac{85}{90} \times 2 = X = \underline{\hspace{1em} 1.9 \hspace{1em}}$

ANSWERS **1.** 2.6 **2.** 1.8 **3.** 0.9 **4.** 1.8 **5.** 1.9

• DECIMAL FRACTIONS •

Equations containing decimal fractions are equally as straightforward to handle.

EXAMPLE 1 $\dfrac{0.3}{1.65} \times 2.5 = X$

$\dfrac{30}{165} \times 2.5$

eliminate the decimal points from the main fraction only

$\dfrac{\cancel{30}^6}{\cancel{165}_{33}} \times 2.5$

reduce the main fraction by dividing by 5

$\dfrac{6 \times 2.5}{33}$

multiply the remaining numerators

$\dfrac{15}{33}$

divide the remaining fraction

X = 0.45 = **0.5**

express to the nearest tenth

EXAMPLE 2 $\dfrac{2.5}{1.5} \times 1.2 = X$

$\dfrac{25}{15} \times 1.2$ eliminate the decimal points from the main fraction

$\dfrac{25^5}{15_3} \times 1.2$ reduce by 5

$\dfrac{6}{3}$ multiply the remaining numerators

$X = 2$ divide the remaining fraction

PROBLEM

Solve the following equations to determine the value of X. Express answers to the nearest tenth.

1. $\dfrac{2.5}{4} \times 1.1 = X = $ _____ .7_____

2. $\dfrac{3.1}{2.7} \times 2.2 = X = $ _____ 2.5 _____

3. $\dfrac{0.05}{1.1} \times 3 = X = $ _____ .1 _____

4. $\dfrac{0.17}{2.2} \times 2.5 = X = $ _____ .2 _____

5. $\dfrac{1.75}{0.95} \times 1.5 = X = $ _____ 2.8 _____

ANSWERS 1. 0.7 2. 2.5 3. 0.1 4. 0.2 5. 2.8

• COMMON FRACTIONS •

Equations containing common fractions are solved as in the following examples.

EXAMPLE 1 $\dfrac{\dfrac{1}{150}}{\dfrac{1}{200}} \times 2 = X$

$\dfrac{1}{150} \times \dfrac{200}{1} \times 2$ invert the fraction representing the denominator

$\dfrac{1}{150_3} \times \dfrac{200^4}{1} \times 2$ reduce the numbers by 50

$$\frac{1}{3} \times \frac{4}{1} \times 2$$ multiply the remaining numerators (4 × 2) and the remaining denominators (3 × 1)

$$\frac{8}{3}$$ divide the remaining fraction

$$X \times 2.66 = \mathbf{2.7}$$ express to the nearest tenth

EXAMPLE 2

$$\frac{\frac{1}{8}}{\frac{1}{6}} \times 2 = X$$ invert the fraction representing the denominator

$$\frac{1}{\cancel{8}_4} \times \frac{\cancel{6}^3}{1} \times 2$$ reduce the numbers by 2

$$\frac{1}{\cancel{4}_2} \times \frac{3}{1} \times \cancel{2}^1$$ reduce again by 2

$$\frac{3}{2}$$ divide the final fraction

$$X = \mathbf{1.5}$$

PROBLEM

Solve the following equations to determine the value of X. Express answers as decimal numbers to the nearest tenth.

1.
$$\frac{\frac{1}{150}}{\frac{1}{100}} \times 2.1 = X = \underline{\quad 1.4 \quad}$$

2.
$$\frac{\frac{1}{8}}{\frac{1}{6}} \times 2.2 = X = \underline{\quad 1.7 \quad}$$

3.
$$\frac{\frac{1}{6}}{\frac{1}{4}} \times 1.4 = X = \underline{\quad .9 \quad}$$

4.
$$\frac{\frac{1}{3}}{\frac{1}{2}} \times 1.2 = X = \underline{\quad .8 \quad}$$

5. $\dfrac{\dfrac{1}{50}}{\dfrac{1}{150}} \times 1.1 = X =$ _____ 3.3

ANSWERS **1.** 1.4   **2.** 1.7   **3.** 0.9   **4.** 0.8   **5.** 3.3

This concludes the refresher on solving equations to determine the value of an unknown X. The important points to remember from this chapter are:

- the first step in solving an equation is to reduce the numbers using common denominators

- the remaining numerators are then multiplied, and divided by the product of the remaining denominators

- answers are expressed as decimal numbers to the nearest tenth

- equations are used for calculations which involve whole numbers, decimal numbers, and common fractions

SUMMARY SELF TEST
Solving For X

DIRECTIONS   Determine the value of X in the following equations. Express your answers as decimal numbers to the nearest tenth.

1. $\dfrac{\dfrac{1}{3}}{\dfrac{1}{5}} \times 1.1 = X =$ _____ 1.8

2. $\dfrac{0.8}{0.65} \times 1.2 = X =$ _____ 1.5

3. $\dfrac{350}{1000} \times 4.4 = X =$ _____ 1.5

4. $\dfrac{\dfrac{1}{200}}{\dfrac{1}{100}} \times 0.7 = X =$ _____ .04

5. $\dfrac{1.3}{0.95} \times 0.5 = X =$ _____ .7

6. $\dfrac{30}{40} \times 3 = X =$ _____ 2.3

7. $\dfrac{1,200,000}{800,000} \times 2.7 = X =$ _____ 4.1

8. $$\frac{\dfrac{3}{4}}{\dfrac{1}{3}} \times 1 \ = X = \underline{\hspace{3cm}}$$

9. $$\frac{0.35}{1.3} \times 4.5 = X = \underline{\hspace{3cm}}$$

10. $$\frac{135}{100} \times 2.5 = X = \underline{\hspace{3cm}} \quad 3.4$$

11. $$\frac{\dfrac{1}{12}}{\dfrac{1}{8}} \times 1.6 = X = \underline{\hspace{3cm}} \quad .8$$

12. $$\frac{0.15}{0.1} \times 1.3 = X = \underline{\hspace{3cm}} \quad 2$$

13. $$\frac{320}{150} \times 1 \ = X = \underline{\hspace{3cm}} \quad 2.1$$

14. $$\frac{0.4}{1.5} \times 2.3 = X = \underline{\hspace{3cm}}$$

15. $$\frac{\dfrac{1}{2}}{\dfrac{1}{4}} \times 1.5 = X = \underline{\hspace{3cm}} \quad 3$$

16. $$\frac{0.08}{0.8} \times 4 \ = X = \underline{\hspace{3cm}}$$

17. $$\frac{20}{15} \times 1.5 = X = \underline{\hspace{3cm}}$$

18. $$\frac{0.003}{0.01} \times 3 \ = X = \underline{\hspace{3cm}}$$

19. $$\frac{1500}{500} \times 0.5 = X = \underline{\hspace{3cm}}$$

20. $$\frac{7.5}{5} \times 2 \ = X = \underline{\hspace{3cm}}$$

ANSWERS

1. 1.8 **2.** 1.5 **3.** 1.5 **4.** 0.4 **5.** 0.7 **6.** 2.3 **7.** 4.1 **8.** 2.3 **9.** 1.2 **10.** 3.4 **11.** 1.1 **12.** 2 **13.** 2.1 **14.** 0.6 **15.** 3
16. 0.4 **17.** 2 **18.** 0.9 **19.** 1.5 **20.** 3

5
Ratio and Proportion

OBJECTIVES
The student will
1. define ratio
2. define proportion
3. define means, and extremes
4. use ratio and proportion to calculate the value of an unknown, X

INTRODUCTION
There are many different ways to calculate drug dosages, but ratio and proportion offers the most logical and safest method of solving any type of dosage or clinical calculation. Once you understand the basic principles of ratio and proportion you will see how simple, yet reliable it is to use. This chapter will review the basics of this method and give you an opportunity to practice using it with a variety of problems. It will also give you a brief introduction to the use of ratio and proportion in setting up and solving actual dosage problems; a topic that will be covered in depth in a later chapter.

• DEFINITION OF RATIO AND PROPORTION •

A ratio is composed of two numbers which are somehow related to each other. These numbers are separated by a colon.

EXAMPLE 1 1 : 50

A ratio can represent any numerical relationship you choose to assign it, but in medications it is used to express the **weight** (strength) of a drug in a **tablet or capsule.**

1 tab : 50 mg (1 tab contains 50 mg of drug)

More commonly in dosage problems, a ratio is used to represent the **weight** of drug **in a certain volume of solution**.

1 mL : 50 mg (1 mL contains 50 mg of drug)

EXAMPLE 2 2 : 500

This ratio, 2 : 500, can be used to represent the following dosage strengths

2 tab contain 500 mg
2 mL contain 500 mg

EXAMPLE 3 A drug which contains 150 mg in 1 mL would be expressed as a ratio by 150 mg : 1 mL (150 : 1)

PROBLEM

Explain what the following ratios mean.

>   **1.** 1.5 mL : 100 mg
>
>   **2.** 0.7 mL : 250 mg
>
>   **3.** 1 tab : 0.4 mg

ANSWERS   **1.** 1.5 mL contain 100 mg of drug   **2.** 0.7 mL contain 250 mg of drug   **3.** 1 tablet contains 0.4 mg of drug

A true proportion consists of two ratios separated by an equal (=) sign or a double colon (::) which indicates that the two ratios are equal. An example of a true proportion would be

$$1 : 50 = 2 : 100$$

This is a simple comparison, and using our previous drug strength example we can mentally verify that the ratios are equal, and the proportion true.

$$1 \text{ tab} : 50 \text{ mg} = 2 \text{ tab} : 100 \text{ mg}$$
$$1 \text{ mL} : 50 \text{ mg} = 2 \text{ mL} : 100 \text{ mg}$$

If 1 tablet contains 50 mg, 2 tablets will contain 100 mg. Similarly if 1 mL contains 50 mg, 2 mL will contain 100 mg.

You can also prove mathematically that these ratios are equal, and that the proportion is true. Look again at the example.

$$1 : 50 = 2 : 100$$

The numbers on the **ends** of the proportion (1, 100) are called the **extremes**, while those in the **middle** (50, 2) are called the **means**.

In a true proportion the product of the means equals the product of the extremes. If you multiply the means, then the extremes, their products (answers) will be equal.

EXAMPLE 1   1 : 50 = 2 : 100

$$\overbrace{1 : \underbrace{50 = 2}_{\text{means}} : 100}^{\text{extremes}}$$

$$50 \times 2 = 100 \times 1$$

$$100 = 100$$

The product of the means, 100, equals the product of the extremes, 100. We have now proved mathematically what we previously proved mentally; the ratios are equal, and the proportion is true.

EXAMPLE 2   2 : 500 = 1 : 250

2 : 500 = 1 : 250

500 × 1 = 2 × 250

500 = 500

The product of the means, 500, equals the product of the extremes, 500. This is a true proportion; the ratios are equal.

   It is critical in all mathematics involving proportions that the means and extremes not be mixed up, or an incorrect answer will be obtained. Here is a memory cue that you can use to prevent confusion. Notice that the **means** are in the **middle** of a proportion. Both of these words begin with an **"m"** (**m**eans, **m**iddle). The **extremes** are on the **ends** of the proportion. Both of these words begin with an **"e"** (**e**xtremes, **e**nds). Use these cues as necessary to prevent mixups.

PROBLEM

Determine mathematically if the following are true proportions.

   1. 34 : 2 = 51 : 3   *True*
   2. 15 : 4 = 45 : 12   *True*
   3. 1.3 : 46 = 0.65 : 23   *True*
   4. 2.3 : 150 = 1.9 : 130 *False*
   5. 40 : 1.1 = 80 : 2.2   *True*
   6. 0.25 : 2 = 0.5 : 4   *True*
   7. 1.5 : 1.4 = 0.75 : 0.7 *True*
   8. 350 : 1 = 700 : 2   *True*
   9. 3.2 : 1.5 = 1.6 : 0.75 *True*
   10. 100 : 1.2 = 75 : 0.4 *False*

ANSWERS   1. True (2 × 51 = 102 and 34 × 3 = 102)   **2.** True (4 × 45 = 180 and 15 × 12 = 180)   **3.** True (1.3 × 23 = 29.9 and 46 × 0.65 = 29.9)   **4.** Not true (2.3 × 130 = 299 and 150 × 1.9 = 285)   **5.** True (40 × 2.2 = 88 and 1.1 × 80 = 88)   **6.** True (0.25 × 4 = 1 and 2 × 0.5 = 1)   **7.** True (1.5 × 0.7 = 1.05 and 1.4 × 0.75 = 1.05)   **8.** True (350 × 2 = 700 and 1 × 700 = 700)   **9.** True (3.2 × 0.75 = 2.4 and 1.5 × 1.6 = 2.4)   **10.** Not true (100 × 0.4 = 40 and 1.2 × 75 = 90)

• USE OF RATIO AND PROPORTION •

Ratio and proportion is important in dosage calculations because it can be used when only one ratio is known, or complete, and the second is incomplete. For example suppose you have a drug with a dosage strength of 8 mg in 1 mL. This gives you a known or complete ratio of 8 mg : 1 mL. However, the doctor orders a dosage of 10 mg. This is your incomplete ratio, and you will use X to represent the unknown mL which will contain 10 mg.

$$8 \text{ mg} : 1 \text{ mL} \quad = \quad 10 \text{ mg} : X \text{ mL}$$

$$\left(\begin{array}{c} \text{complete ratio} \\ \text{drug strength} \end{array} \right) \quad \left(\begin{array}{c} \text{incomplete ratio} \\ \text{dosage to give} \end{array} \right)$$

The major precaution in setting up the proportion is that **the ratios must be written in the same sequence of measurement units**. In the above example they are

$$\text{mg} : \text{mL} = \text{mg} : \text{mL}$$

Next let's look at the math steps used to determine the value of X

EXAMPLE 1 $8 \text{ mg} : 1 \text{ mL} = 10 \text{ mg} : X \text{ mL}$ check sequence of measurement units; mg : mL = mg : mL

$8 : 1 = 10 : X$ drop the measurement units

$10 = 8X$ multiply the means, then the extremes

$\dfrac{10}{8} = X$ divide 10 by the number in front of X

$\dfrac{\cancel{10}^{5}}{\cancel{8}_{4}} = X$ reduce the numbers by 2, divide the final fraction

$X = 1.25$ **the unknown, X, is 1.25 mL**

To give the ordered dosage of 10 mg you must administer 1.25 mL. It is routine to check your math twice in dosage calculations. However, it is also necessary to **assess each answer to determine if it seems logical**. Here is where our previous review of relative value of numbers is put to use. Consider the answer you just obtained in example 1.

$$8 \text{ mg} : 1 \text{ mL} = 10 \text{ mg} : X \text{ mL}$$

$$X = 1.25 \text{ mL}$$

If **1 mL** contains **8 mg** you will need a **larger** volume then 1 mL to obtain **10 mg**. The answer you obtained, 1.25 mL, **is** larger, therefore it is logical. This routine check does not guarantee that your math is correct, but it does indicate that you have not mixed up the means and extremes in your calculations.

You can prove that the proportion is true (and your math correct) by substituting your answer for X in the original proportion.

$$8 \text{ mg} : 1 \text{ mL} = 10 \text{ mg} : X \text{ mL}$$

$$8 \text{ mg} : 1 \text{ mL} = 10 \text{ mg} : 1.25 \text{ mL}$$

$$10 = 8 \times 1.25$$

$$10 = 10$$

You have now proved mathematically that your answer is correct. However, in most routine calculations it is neither necessary nor practical to mathematically prove each answer you obtain. Dosages such as the 1.25 mL in our example are routinely rounded off to the nearest tenth (1.25 = 1.3 mL). Once this is done, the math proofing the answer may contain small discrepancies that could cause confusion.

EXAMPLE 2   The strength available is 25 mg in 1.5 mL. A dosage of 20 mg has been ordered.

25 mg : 1.5 mL = 20 mg : X mL   make sure the units are in
the same sequence:
mg : mL = mg : mL

25 : 1.5 = 20 : X   drop the measurement units

1.5 × 20 = 25X   multiply the means, then the
extremes

$$\frac{30}{25} = X$$ divide by the number in front of X

$$\frac{30^6}{25_5} = 1.2$$ reduce by 5, and divide the final fraction

X = **1.2 mL**

Your routine check indicates that X should be a smaller number than 1.5 mL (20 mg is less than 25 mg), and it is (1.2 mL is smaller than 1.5 mL).

These examples will give you an idea of how ratio and proportion is used to solve dosage problems. However, our focus in this chapter is the math involved in this skill, and the balance of the chapter will focus entirely on math. A later chapter will cover actual dosage problems in depth.

EXAMPLE 3   100 : 2 = 80 : X

2 × 80 = 100X

$$\frac{160}{100} = X$$

$$\frac{16^8}{10_5} = X = \mathbf{1.6}$$

80 is a smaller quantity than 100, and the answer you obtain must be smaller than 2, which it is (1.6).

PROBLEM

Determine the value of X in the following proportions. Practice proofing your answers mathematically.

1. 12.5 : 5 = 24 : X   9.6

2. 40 : 2.5 = 30 : X   1.9

3. 0.6 : 0.8 = 0.3 : X   .4

4. 36 : 2 = 24 : X   1.3

5. 78 : 0.9 = 52 : X   .6

ANSWERS **1.** 9.6 **2.** 1.9 **3.** 0.4 **4.** 1.3 **5.** 0.6

Ratio and proportion works equally as well with common fractions.

EXAMPLE 1 $\frac{1}{2} : 2 = \frac{1}{8} : X$

$2 \times \frac{1}{8} = \frac{1}{2}X$ multiply the means, then the extremes

$\dfrac{2 \times \frac{1}{8}}{\frac{1}{2}} = X$ divide by the number in front of X

$2 \times \frac{1}{8} \times \frac{2}{1} = X$ convert the denominator $\frac{1}{2}$

to an equivalent multiplication $\frac{2}{1}$

$\cancel{2}^1 \times \frac{1}{\cancel{8}_{\,2}} \times \cancel{2}^1 = X$ reduce

$X = \frac{1}{2} = \mathbf{0.5}$ divide the final fraction

Your answer should be smaller, $\frac{1}{8}$ is less than $\frac{1}{2}$, and it is (0.5 is less than 2).

EXAMPLE 2 $\frac{1}{4} : 1.5 = \frac{1}{2} : X$

$1.5 \times \frac{1}{2} = \frac{1}{4}X$

$\dfrac{1.5 \times \frac{1}{2}}{\frac{1}{4}} = X$

$1.5 \times \frac{1}{\cancel{2}_1} \times \frac{\cancel{4}^2}{1} = X = \mathbf{3}$

Your answer should be larger than 1.5 because $\frac{1}{2}$ is a larger quantity than $\frac{1}{4}$,

and it is.

PROBLEM

Determine the value of X in the following proportions. Proof each of your answers mathematically.

1. $\frac{1}{2} : 2 = \frac{1}{8} : X$ .5

2. $\frac{1}{75} : 4 = \frac{1}{100} : X$ 3.3 ?

3. $\frac{1}{4} : 1.6 = \frac{1}{8} : X$ .8

4. $\frac{1}{5} : 1.8 = \frac{1}{4} : X$ 2.

5. $\frac{1}{100} : 1.3 = \frac{1}{150} : X$

ANSWERS 1. 0.5 **2.** 3 **3.** 0.8 **4.** 2.3 **5.** 0.9

As soon as you are comfortable with the math steps in ratio and proportion you can combine several steps at once, and work even more efficiently. Look at the combined steps in the following examples.

EXAMPLE 1 $300 : 1.2 = 120 : X$ set up the proportion with the known ratio written first

$$\frac{1.2 \times 120}{300} = X$$ multiply the means, and **immediately** divide by the number in front of X

$$\frac{1.2 \times \cancel{120}^{2}}{\cancel{300}_{5}} = \frac{2.4}{5} = 0.48 = \mathbf{0.5}$$ reduce, do final math

Check your answer; 120 is a smaller quantity than 300, and your answer, **0.5**, is smaller than 1.2, as it should be.

EXAMPLE 2 $3.5 : 1.7 = 5.1 : X$

$$\frac{1.7 \times 5.1}{3.5} = X = 2.47 = \mathbf{2.5}$$

The quantity, 5.1, is larger than 3.5, so the answer, 2.5, must also be larger than 1.7, and it is.

EXAMPLE 3 $\frac{1}{150} : 2 = \frac{1}{100} : X$

$$2 \times \frac{1}{100} \times \frac{150}{1} = X$$ change the common fraction representing the divisor immediately to convert to a multiplication

$$2^1 \times \frac{1}{\cancel{100}_2} \times \frac{\cancel{150}^3}{1} = 3$$

$\frac{1}{100}$ is a larger quantity than $\frac{1}{150}$ and your answer, 3, is also larger (than 2).

This concludes the introductory chapter on ratio and proportion. The important points to remember from this chapter are:

- a ratio is composed of two numbers that are somehow related to each other

- a proportion consists of two ratios which are equal to each other

- if one number of a proportion is missing it can be determined mathematically by multiplying the means, and the extremes, and solving the equation

- when ratio and proportion is used to solve dosage problems the critical first step is to set the ratios up in the same sequence of measurement units

- the math of calculations must always be double checked and the answer must be assessed logically to determine if X is appropriately larger or smaller than the strength available.

SUMMARY SELF TEST
Ratio and Proportion

DIRECTIONS Determine the value of X in the following proportions. Express fractional answers as decimal fractions to the nearest tenth.

1. $75 : 5 = 187.5 : X$ = _____12.5_____

2. $7500 : 1.5 = 10,000 : X$ = _____

3. $17 : 3 = 42.5 : X$ = _____

4. $0.25 : 0.8 = 0.75 : X$ = _____

5. $55 : 1.1 = 165 : X$ = _____3.3_____

6. $14.2 : 1.3 = 12.1 : X$ = _____

7. $250 : 2.3 = 325 : X$ = _____

8. $40 : 1 = 30 : X$ = _____

9. $12.5 : 1.2 = 6.25 : X$ = _____

10. $200,000 : 2.5 = 150,000 : X$ = _____1.9_____

11. $0.02 : 1.2 = 0.05 : X$ = _____

12. $125 : 0.8 = 100 : X$ = _____

13. $350 : 1.6 = 175 : X$ = _____

14. $1250 : 1.4 = 625 : X$ = _____

15. $175 : 0.6 = 225 : X$ = _____.8_____

16. $750 : 1.5 = 1125 : X$ = _____

17. $0.7 : 1.2 = 0.8 : X$ = _____

18. $0.04 : 0.5 = 0.12 : X$ = _____

19. $\frac{1}{10} : 1.8 = \frac{1}{12} : X$ = _____

20. $\frac{1}{2} : 1.4 = \frac{1}{3} : X$ = ___.9___

21. $\frac{1}{6} : 2 = \frac{1}{10} : X$ = _____

22. $7.5 : 3.2 = 10 : X$ = _____

23. $100,000 : 2 = 75,000 : X$ = _____

24. $0.1 : 0.3 = 0.25 : X$ = _____

25. $\frac{1}{50} : 1.1 = \frac{1}{75} : X$ = _____

26. $\frac{1}{200} : 1.4 = \frac{1}{150} : X$ = _____

27. $\frac{1}{4} : 1.8 = \frac{1}{3} : X$ = _____

28. $15.7 : 2.3 = 14.2 : X$ = _____

29. $45 : 1.2 = 35 : X$ = _____

30. $275 : 2.3 = 250 : X$ = ___2.1___

ANSWERS

1. 12.5   2. 2   3. 7.5   4. 2.4   5. 3.3   6. 1.1   7. 3   8. 0.8   9. 0.6   10. 1.9   11. 3   12. 0.6   13. 0.8   14. 0.7   15. 0.8   16. 2.3   17. 1.4   18. 1.5   19. 1.5   20. 0.9   21. 1.2   22. 4.3   23. 1.5   24. 0.8   25. 0.7   26. 1.9   27. 2.4   28. 2.1   29. 0.9   30. 2.1

6

Equivalents in Decimals, Common Fractions, Ratios, and Percents

OBJECTIVES
The student will
1. define percentage solution
2. explain the relationship between decimals, common fractions, ratios, and percents
3. express decimals, common fractions, ratios and percents as equivalents of each other

INTRODUCTION
In previous chapters we have reviewed the math of decimals, common fractions, and ratios. In this chapter we will add an additional measure, percents. Drug dosages are expressed using all of these measures: for example you may see 1 : 1000 (a ratio); grains ¼ (a common fraction); 0.25 grams (a decimal); and 1% (a percentage). All of these measures can be expressed as equivalents of each other.

• DEFINITION OF PERCENT •

Percent (%) means **parts per hundred**. In medications percent is used to express the **number of grams of drug per 100 mL/cc of solvent**.

EXAMPLE 1   100 mL of a 1% solution will contain 1 gram of drug

EXAMPLE 2   100 mL of a 2% solution will contain 2 grams of drug

EXAMPLE 3   50 mL of a 1% solution will contain 0.5 grams of drug

EXAMPLE 4   200 mL of a 2% solution will contain 4 grams of drug

PROBLEM

1. How many grams of drug will 100 mL of a 10% solution contain? _____

2. How many grams of drug will 50 mL of a 10% solution contain? _____

3. How many grams of drug will 200 mL of a 10% solution contain? _____

ANSWERS   **1.** 10 grams   **2.** 5 grams   **3.** 20 grams

Calculating the number of grams of drug in a percentage solution is occasionally necessary in intravenous fluid administration. For the present however, it is simply necessary for you to remember that percent means parts per hundred.

• CONVERTING BETWEEN RATIOS AND COMMON FRACTIONS •

The easiest of the conversions to do is between ratios and common fractions, because they are essentially the same. Refer to figure 7 and notice how the colon of the ratio (:), and the fraction bar (—) of the common fraction both serve to identify the numerator and denominator of these two measures.

$$7 : 100 \qquad\qquad \frac{7}{100} \quad \text{numerator} \atop \text{denominator}$$

numerator   denominator

Figure 7

Conversion from ratio to common fraction, and vice versa, requires just a physical realignment of the numbers.

EXAMPLE 1 $2 : 5 = \dfrac{2}{5}$

EXAMPLE 2 $\dfrac{1}{10} = 1 : 10$

PROBLEM

Convert the following ratios and common fractions to their equivalents.

	Ratio	Common Fraction
1.	1 : 2	½
2.	3 : 4	3/4
3.	2 : 5	$\dfrac{2}{5}$
4.	1 : 6	$\dfrac{1}{6}$

ANSWERS   1. $\dfrac{1}{2}$ 2. $\dfrac{3}{4}$ 3. 2 : 5   4. 1 : 6

• CHANGING RATIOS, COMMON FRACTIONS AND DECIMALS TO PERCENT •

If it is necessary to express a decimal, ratio or common fraction as a percent, you must simply multiply by 100. **Percent is always obtained by multiplying by 100 and adding the % sign.** Ratios and common fractions are converted by changing ratios to common fractions first, because the physical alignment of the numbers is easier to work with.

EXAMPLE 1
$$1 : 4 = \frac{1}{\cancel{4}_1} \times \cancel{100}^{25} = 25\%$$

EXAMPLE 2
$$2 : 5 = \frac{2}{\cancel{5}_1} \times \cancel{100}^{20} = 40\%$$

EXAMPLE 3
$$1 : 6 = \frac{1}{6} \times 100 = 16.67 = 16.7\%$$

Round off to the nearest tenth percent

EXAMPLE 4
$$1 : 100 = \frac{1}{100} \times 100 = 1\%$$

Notice that **when the denominator is 100**, as in example 4, **the percent equivalent is always the same as the original numerator** ($\frac{1}{100} = 1\%$). Therefore if the denominator is 100, the conversion is already done: the percent equivalent is the same as the numerator.

EXAMPLE 5
$$3 : 100 = \frac{3}{\cancel{100}_1} \times \cancel{100}^1 = 3\%$$

PROBLEM

Express the following ratios as common fractions, then as percentage equivalents.

	Ratio	Common Fraction	%
1.	3 : 4	3/4	75
2.	1 : 8	1/4	12.5
3.	1 : 1000	1/1000	.01
4.	3 : 10	3/10	30
5.	0.9 : 100	.9/100	.9

ANSWERS   **1.** $\frac{3}{4}$, 75%   **2.** $\frac{1}{8}$, 12.5%   **3.** $\frac{1}{1000}$, 0.1%   **4.** $\frac{3}{10}$, 30%   **5.** $\frac{0.9}{100}$, 0.9%

To convert a decimal to a percent it is also necessary to **multiply by 100.** However, in decimal numbers this is done by simply moving the decimal point. **The number of places the decimal point is moved is the same as the number of zeros in the multiplier.** For 100, this is 2 places. **When you multiply, the quantity must get larger, so the decimal point is moved two places to the right.** Zeros may need to be eliminated or added to accomplish this.

Decimal	Percent

EXAMPLE 1   0.02   2%

Move the decimal point in 0.02 two places to the right making it 2. One zero is eliminated.

EXAMPLE 2   0.001   0.1%

Two zeros are dropped

EXAMPLE 3   0.3   30%

One zero is added

PROBLEM

Convert the following decimals to percents.

1. 0.4   = ___40 %___
2. 0.05 = ___5 %___
3. 0.25 = ___25 %___
4. 0.004 = ___.4 %___
5. 0.15 = ___15 %___

ANSWERS **1.** 40% **2.** 5% **3.** 25% **4.** 0.4% **5.** 15%

Special Note: All multiplications (and divisions) by units of 10 (10, 100, 1000) can be done by moving the decimal point. The number of places the decimal point is moved is always the same as the number of zeros in the multiplier (or divider). For 10, this is one place; for 100 it is two places; for 1000 it is three places.

• CONVERTING PERCENT TO DECIMALS, COMMON FRACTIONS, AND RATIOS •

When you wish to reverse these conversions and **change percent back to the other measures you must divide by 100**. The conversion of a **percent to a decimal** once again is accomplished by **moving the decimal point**. Because you are dividing by 100 the quantity will get smaller, and the decimal point will move two places to the left.

	Percent	**Decimal**
EXAMPLE 1	7%	0.07
EXAMPLE 2	25%	0.25
EXAMPLE 3	0.1%	0.001
EXAMPLE 4	0.02%	0.0002

PROBLEM

Change the following percents to decimal equivalents.

1. 20%   = ___.20___
2. 0.5% = ___.005___
3. 2.5% = ___.025___

4. 0.08% = ___.0008___

5. 4%   = ___.04___

ANSWERS   **1.** 0.2   **2.** 0.005   **3.** 0.025   **4.** 0.0008   **5.** 0.04

To convert from percent to common fractions and ratios make the common fraction conversion first.

		Common Fraction	Ratio
EXAMPLE 1	3%	$\dfrac{3}{100}$	3 : 100
EXAMPLE 2	1%	$\dfrac{1}{100}$	1 : 100
EXAMPLE 3	2%	$\dfrac{2}{100}$	2 : 100

$\dfrac{2}{100}$ can be reduced to its lowest terms and expressed as $\dfrac{1}{50}$, 1 : 50

		Common Fraction	Ratio
EXAMPLE 4	25%	$\dfrac{25}{100}$	25 : 100
		or $\dfrac{1}{4}$	1 : 4
EXAMPLE 5	0.9%	$\dfrac{0.9}{100}$	0.9 : 100

The 0.9 can also be expressed as a whole number ratio or fraction by eliminating the decimal point.

$\dfrac{0.9}{100}$ becomes $\dfrac{9}{1000}$ and 9 : 1000

		Common Fraction	Ratio
EXAMPLE 6	0.01%	$\dfrac{0.01}{100}$	0.01 : 100
		$\dfrac{1}{10,000}$	1 : 10,000

PROBLEM

Express the following percents as common fractions and ratios. Reduce the equivalents to their lowest terms, and express decimal fraction strengths as whole numbers.

Percent	Common Fraction	Ratio
1. 4%	4/100 (1/25)	4 : 100 (r = 25)
2. 10%	10/100 ? 1/10	1 : 10

      3. 2.5%   _____   _____

      4. 0.5%   _____   _____

      5. 0.02%   _____   _____

ANSWERS   **1.** $\frac{1}{25}$, 1 : 25   **2.** $\frac{1}{10}$, 1 : 10   **3.** $\frac{1}{40}$, 1 : 40   **4.** $\frac{1}{200}$, 1 : 200   **5.** $\frac{1}{5,000}$, 1 : 5,000

• CHANGING DECIMALS TO COMMON FRACTIONS AND RATIOS •

To change a decimal fraction to a common fraction or ratio you must first recognize that **a decimal fraction has an unwritten denominator of 10, or a multiple of 10 (100, 1000). Identify the denominator by looking at the position of the decimal point.**

EXAMPLE 1   0.3 is the same as $\frac{3}{10}$ 3 : 10

One number after the decimal identifies tenths.

EXAMPLE 2 $0.01 = \frac{1}{100}$ 1 : 100

Two numbers after the decimal identifies hundredths.

EXAMPLE 3 $0.015 = \frac{15}{1000}$ 15 : 1000

Three numbers after the decimal point identifies thousandths. This fraction/ratio can also be reduced to its lowest terms, and expressed as $\frac{3}{200}$, 3 : 200

PROBLEM

Change the following decimal fractions to their common fraction and ratio equivalents. Reduce to lowest terms.

Decimal Fraction	Common Fraction	Ratio
1. 0.9	$^9/_{10}$	9 : 10
2. 0.75	$^{75}/_{100}$	75 : 100 3=4
3. 0.01	$^1/_{100}$	1 : 100
4. 0.45	$^{45}/_{100}$ $^9/_{20}$	9 : 20
5. 0.003	$^3/_{1000}$	3 : 1000

ANSWERS   **1.** $\frac{9}{10}$, 9 : 10   **2.** $\frac{3}{4}$, 3 : 4   **3.** $\frac{1}{100}$, 1 : 100   **4.** $\frac{9}{20}$, 9 : 20   **5.** $\frac{3}{1000}$, 3 : 1000

• CHANGING RATIOS AND COMMON FRACTIONS TO DECIMAL EQUIVALENTS •

The last equivalent that must be covered is one you have already practiced in previous chapters. **To change a ratio or common fraction to a decimal you must divide the numerator by the denominator.**

	Ratio	Common Fraction	Decimal Fraction
EXAMPLE 1	2 : 5	$\frac{2}{5}$	0.4
EXAMPLE 2	3 : 4	$\frac{3}{4}$	0.75
EXAMPLE 3	2 : 3	$\frac{2}{3}$	0.666 = 0.67

PROBLEM

Convert the following ratios to common fractions, then to decimal fractions. Round to the nearest hundredth.

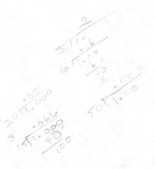

	Ratio	Common Fraction	Decimal Fraction
1.	1 : 5	$\frac{1}{5}$	.2
2.	1 : 6	$\frac{1}{6}$	.17
3.	1 : 50	$\frac{1}{50}$	.02
4.	1 : 20	$\frac{1}{20}$	.05
5.	1 : 15	$\frac{1}{15}$	.07

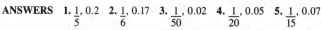

ANSWERS   **1.** $\frac{1}{5}$, 0.2   **2.** $\frac{1}{6}$, 0.17   **3.** $\frac{1}{50}$, 0.02   **4.** $\frac{1}{20}$, 0.05   **5.** $\frac{1}{15}$, 0.07

This concludes the chapter on equivalents in drug measures. The important points to remember are:

- dosages may be expressed as ratios, percents, common fractions, or decimal fractions

- all of these measures can be expressed as equivalents of each other

- ratios and common fractions are essentially the same, with only the colon or fraction bar making then look different

- to change a percent to any other equivalent divide by 100

- to change any other equivalent to a percent multiply by 100

- to change a common fraction or ratio to a decimal fraction divide the numerator by the denominator

- to reverse this calculation, and express a decimal fraction as a common fraction or ratio, write the appropriate denominator beneath the decimal fraction and reduce to simplest terms

Equivalents in Decimals, Common Fractions, Ratios and Percents

DIRECTIONS Express each of the following measures as their three mathematic equivalents. Reduce to simplest terms where appropriate.

Percent	Ratio	Common Fraction	Decimal
1. 0.01%	1 : 1000	$\frac{1}{1000}$	.0001
2. .02%	1 : 2000	$\frac{1}{2000}$	.0002
3.	1 : 25	$\frac{1}{25}$	
4.			0.02
5. 10%			
6.		$\frac{1}{3}$	
7.		$\frac{1}{150}$	
8.			0.15
9.			0.03
10. 0.45%			
11.		$\frac{1}{4}$	
12.	1 : 100		
13.			0.06
14. 2.5%			
15. 20%			
16.		$\frac{1}{2}$	
17.			0.9
18.	1 : 200		
19.	1 : 15		
20.		$\frac{3}{50}$	

ANSWERS

	Percent	Ratio	Common Fraction	Decimal Fraction
1.	**0.01%**	1 : 10,000	$\dfrac{1}{10,000}$	0.0001
2.	0.05%	**1 : 2000**	$\dfrac{1}{2,000}$	0.0005
3.	4%	**1 : 25**	$\dfrac{1}{25}$	0.04
4.	2%	1 : 50	$\dfrac{1}{50}$	**0.02**
5.	**10%**	1 : 10	$\dfrac{1}{10}$	0.1
6.	33.3%	1 : 3	$\dfrac{\mathbf{1}}{\mathbf{3}}$	0.33
7.	0.67%	1 : 150	$\dfrac{\mathbf{1}}{\mathbf{150}}$	0.0067
8.	15%	3 : 20	$\dfrac{3}{20}$	**0.15**
9.	3%	3 : 100	$\dfrac{3}{100}$	**0.03**
10.	**0.45%**	9 : 2000	$\dfrac{9}{2000}$	0.0045
11.	25%	1 : 4	$\dfrac{\mathbf{1}}{\mathbf{4}}$	0.25
12.	1%	**1 : 100**	$\dfrac{1}{100}$	0.01
13.	6%	3 : 50	$\dfrac{3}{50}$	**0.06**
14.	**2.5%**	1 : 40	$\dfrac{1}{40}$	0.025
15.	**20%**	1 : 5	$\dfrac{1}{5}$	0.2
16.	50%	1 : 2	$\dfrac{\mathbf{1}}{\mathbf{2}}$	0.5
17.	90%	9 : 10	$\dfrac{9}{10}$	**0.9**
18.	0.5%	**1 : 200**	$\dfrac{1}{200}$	0.005
19.	6.7%	**1 : 15**	$\dfrac{1}{15}$	0.067
20.	6%	3 : 50	$\dfrac{\mathbf{3}}{\mathbf{50}}$	0.06

SECTION
TWO

Systems of
Drug Measure

7

The Metric/SI/International System

OBJECTIVES
The student will
1. list the commonly used units of measure in the metric system
2. distinguish between the official abbreviations and variations in common use
3. express metric weights and volumes using correct notation rules
4. convert metric weights and volumes within the system

INTRODUCTION
The major system of weights and measures used in medicine is the metric/international/SI (from the French **S**ystème **I**nternational). The metric system was invented in France in 1875, and takes its name from the **meter**, a length roughly equivalent to a yard, from which all other units of measure in the system are derived. The strength of the metric system lies in its simplicity, since all units of measure differ from each other in powers of ten (10). Conversions between units in the system are accomplished by simply moving a decimal point.

While it is not necessary for you to know the entire metric system to administer medications safely, you must understand its basic structure, and become familiar with the units of measure you will be using.

• BASIC UNITS OF METRIC MEASURE •

Three types of metric measures are in common use, those for length, volume (or capacity), and weight. The basic units or beginning points of these three measures are

length ———— meter

volume ———— liter

weight ———— gram

You must memorize these basic units: do so now if you do not already know them. In addition to these basic units there are both larger and smaller units of measure for length, volume, and weight. Let's compare this concept with something familiar. The pound is a unit of weight that we use every day. A smaller unit of measure is the ounce, a larger, the ton. **All are units measuring weight.**

In the same way there are smaller and larger units than the basic meter, liter, and gram. However, in the metric system there is one very important advantage: **all other units, whether larger or smaller than the basic units, have the name of the basic unit incorporated in them**. So there is never need for doubt when you see a unit of measure just what it is measuring. **Meter-length, liter-volume, gram-weight.**

PROBLEM

Identify the following metric measures with their appropriate category of weight, length, or volume.

1. milligram _____weight_____
2. centimeter _____length_____
3. milliliter _____volume_____
4. millimeter _____length_____
5. kilogram _____weight_____
6. microgram _____weight_____

ANSWERS 1. weight 2. length 3. volume 4. length 5. weight 6. weight

• METRIC PREFIXES •

The prefixes used in combination with the names of the basic units identify the larger and smaller units of measure. The same prefixes are used with all three measures. Therefore there is a kilo**meter**, kilo**gram**, and a kilo**liter**. Prefixes also change the value of each of the basic units by the same amount. For example the prefix "kilo" identifies a unit of measure which is larger than, or multiplies the basic unit by 1000. Therefore,

    1 kilometer = 1000 meters
    1 kilogram = 1000 grams
    1 kiloliter = 1000 liters

Kilo is the only prefix you will be using which identifies a measure **larger** than the basic unit. Kilograms are frequently used as a measure for body weight, especially for infants and children.

You will see only three measures **smaller** than the basic unit in common use. The prefixes for these are:

        centi — as in centimeter
        milli — as in milligram
        micro — as in microgram

Therefore, you will actually be working with only four prefixes; kilo, which identifies a larger unit of measure than the basics, and centi, milli, and micro, which identify smaller units than the basics.

• METRIC ABBREVIATIONS •

In actual use the units of measure are abbreviated. **The basic units are abbreviated to their first initial, and printed in small letters, with the exception of liter which is capitalized.** Therefore,

        gram is g
        meter is m
        liter is L

The abbreviations for the prefixes used in combination with the basic units are all printed using small letters.

kilo ——— k ——— as in kilogram ——— kg
centi ——— c ——— as in centimeter ——— cm
milli ——— m ——— as in milligram ——— mg
micro ——— mc ——— as in microgram ——— mcg

Micro has an additional abbreviation, the symbol µ, which is used in combination with the basic unit, as in microgram, µg.

While you will see the symbol µg on drug labels for microgram, you should be aware that it has an inherent safety risk. When hand printed it is very easy for microgram (*mg*) to be mistaken for milligram (*mg*). These units differ from each other in value by 1000 (1 mg = 1000 mcg), and misreading these dosages could be critical.

To assure safety when transcribing orders by hand always use the abbreviation mc to designate micro rather than its symbol: Example mcg.

In combination liter remains capitalized. Therefore milliliter is mL, and kiloliter kL.

PROBLEM

Print the abbreviations for the following metric units.

1. microgram _____mcg_____
2. liter _____L_____
3. kilogram _____kg_____
4. milliliter _____mL_____
5. centimeter _____cm_____
6. milligram _____mg_____
7. meter _____m_____
8. kiloliter _____kL_____
9. millimeter _____mm_____
10. gram _____g_____

ANSWERS   1. mcg   2. L   3. kg   4. mL   5. cm   6. mg   7. m   8. kL   9. mm   10. g

• VARIATIONS OF SI/METRIC ABBREVIATIONS •

Although the metric system was invented in 1875 it was not until 1960, nearly 100 years later, that a standard system of abbreviations, the **International System of Units**, was adopted. Therefore a variety of unofficial abbreviations are still in use. Most of the variations were designed to prevent confusion with the much older apothecaries' system, which was in common use at that time in drug dosages. The major difference is that gram was abbreviated **Gm**, in an effort to differentiate it from the apothecaries' grain, **gr**. This of course led to milligram and microgram being abbreviated **mgm**, and **mcgm**. Liter was routinely abbreviated small **l**, and milliliter, **ml**. While you may see these abbreviations on occasion do not fall into the habit of using them. They are officially obsolete.

• METRIC NOTATION RULES •

The easiest way to learn the rules of metric notations in which a unit of measure is expressed with a quantity, is to memorize some prototypes (examples) which incorporate all the rules. Then if you get confused, you can stop and think and remember the correct way to write them. For the metric system the notations for one-half, one, and one and one-half milliliters will incorporate all the rules you must know.

0.5 mL   **1 mL**   **1.5 mL**

RULES: The quantity is written in Arabic numerals, 1,2,3,4, etc.

EXAMPLE 0.5 1 1.5

- **The numerals representing the quantity are placed in front of the abbreviations.**

EXAMPLE 0.5 mL 1 mL 1.5 mL (not mL 0.5, etc.)

- **A full space is used between the numeral and abbreviation.**

EXAMPLE 0.5 mL 1 mL 1.5 mL (not 0.5mL, etc.)

- **Fractional parts of a unit are expressed as decimal fractions.**

EXAMPLE 0.5 mL 1.5 mL (not ½ mL, 1½ mL)

- **A zero is placed in front of the decimal when it is not preceded by a whole number to emphasize the decimal point.**

EXAMPLE 0.5 mL (not .5 mL)

- **Unnecessary zeros are omitted so they cannot be misread and lead to medication errors.**

EXAMPLE 0.5 mL 1 mL 1.5 mL (not 0.50 mL, 1.0 mL, 1.50 mL)

So once again, as examples of the rules of metric notations, memorize the prototypes 0.5 mL–1 mL–1.5 mL. Just refer back to these in your memory if you get confused and you will be able to write them correctly.

PROBLEM

Write the following metric measures using official abbreviations and notation rules.

1. two grams . . . . _2.0 g_
2. five hundred milliliters . . . . _500 mL_
3. five-tenths of a liter . . . . _.5 L_
4. two-tenths of a milligram . . . . _.2 mg_
5. five-hundredths of a gram . . . . _.05 g_
6. two and five tenths kilograms . . . . _2.5 kg_
7. one hundred micrograms . . . . _100 mcg_

8. two and three-tenths milliliters. . . . . _2.3 mL_
9. seven-tenths of a milliliter . . . . _.7 mL_
10. three-tenths of a milligram. . . . . _.3 mg_
11. two and four tenths liters . . . . _2.4 L_
12. seventeen and five-tenths kilograms. . . . . . _17.5 kg_
13. nine-hundredths of a milligram . . . . _.09 mg_
14. ten and two-tenths micrograms . . . . _10.2 mcg_
15. four-hundredths of a gram . . . . _.04 g_

ANSWERS   1. 2 g   **2.** 500 mL   **3.** 0.5 L   **4.** 0.2 mg   **5.** 0.05 g   **6.** 2.5 kg   **7.** 100 mcg   **8.** 2.3 mL
9. 0.7 mL   **10.** 0.3 mg   **11.** 2.4 L   **12.** 17.5 kg   **13.** 0.09 mg   **14.** 10.2 mcg   **15.** 0.04 g

---

• CONVERSION BETWEEN METRIC/SI UNITS •

When you administer medications you will routinely be converting units of measure within the metric system, for example g to mg, and mg to mcg. Learning the relative value of the units you will be working with is the first prerequisite to accurate conversions. There are only four metric **weights** commonly used in medicine. From **highest** to **lowest** value these are:

        kg   = kilogram
        g   = gram
        mg   = milligram
        mcg   = microgram

Only two units of **volume** are frequently used. From **highest** to **lowest** value these are:

        L   = liter
        mL   = milliliter

Each of these units differs in value from the next by 1000

        1 kg = 1000 g
        1 g   = 1000 mg
        1 mg = 1000 mcg

        1 L   = 1000 mL (1000 cc)

The abbreviations for milliliter (mL) and cubic centimeter (cc) are used interchangeably. A cc is actually the amount of physical space that a 1 mL volume occupies, but the two measures are considered identical.

Once again, from highest to lowest value the units are, for weight: kg—g—mg—mcg; for volume: L—mL (cc). Each unit differs in value from the next by 1000, and **all conversions will be between touching units of measure**, for example g to mg, mg to mcg, L to mL.

PROBLEM

Indicate if the following statements are true or false.

        1. T   F   1000 cc   = 1000 L

2.	T	F	1000 mg	= 1 g	T
3.	T	F	1000 mL	= 1000 cc	T
4.	T	F	1000 mg	= 1 mcg	F
5.	T	F	1000 mcg	= 1 g	F
6.	T	F	1 kg	= 1000 g	T
7.	T	F	1 mg	= 1000 g	F
8.	T	F	1000 mcg	= 1 mg	T
9.	T	F	1000 mL	= 1 L	T
10.	T	F	3 cc	= 3 mL	T

Handwritten: $1 g = $ 1 millionth of g should be $\left(\frac{1000}{1000} = \frac{1000000}{1000000}\right)$ to be T

$\frac{1000}{1000} = \frac{1}{1000000}$

$\frac{1000}{1000000} = \frac{1}{1000}$ *$\frac{1000}{1000000} = \frac{1}{1000}$ True*

ANSWERS 1. F 2. T 3. T 4. F 5. F 6. T 7. F 8. T 9. T 10. T

Since the metric system is a decimal system, conversions between the units are simply a matter of moving the decimal point. Also because each unit of measure in common use differs from the next by 1000, if you know one conversion you know them all.

How far do you move the decimal point? Each of the units differs from the next by 1000. There are three zeros in 1000, **move the decimal point three places**.

Which way do you move the decimal point? If you are converting **down** the scale to a **smaller** unit of measure, for example g to mg, the quantity must get larger, so move the decimal three places to the **right**.

EXAMPLE 1 0.5 g = __500__ mg

Handwritten: $\frac{1}{1000}$ .5 .5 000

You are converting down the scale. Move the decimal point three places to the right. To do this you have to add two zeros. Your answer, 500 mg, is a larger number because you moved down the scale (0.5 g = 500 mg).

EXAMPLE 2 2.5 L = __2500__ mL   *2.5 000*

Converting down, L to mL, move the decimal point three places to the right. Your answer will be a larger quantity (2.5 L = 2500 mL).

PROBLEM

Handwritten: 1500 mg = 1.5 g

Convert the following metric measures

Handwritten: 7000

1.	7 mg	= __7000__	mcg
2.	1.7 L	= __1700__	mL
3.	3.2 g	= __3200__	mg
4.	0.03 kg	= __30__	g
5.	0.4 mg	= __400__	mcg
6.	1.5 mg	= __1500__	mcg
7.	0.7 g	= __700__	mg
8.	0.3 L	= __300__	mL
9.	7 kg	= __7000__	g

Handwritten: 1,700

Handwritten: 1000 > 1000000

Handwritten: $\underset{10}{1} < \underset{100}{1} < \underset{1000}{1} < 10000$

Handwritten: ×1000 4,000

Handwritten: Bigger   Smaller

10. 0.01 mg = _____110_____ mcg

ANSWERS   **1.** 7000 mcg   **2.** 1700 mL   **3.** 3200 mg   **4.** 30 g   **5.** 400 mcg   **6.** 1500 mcg   **7.** 700 mg   **8.** 30 mL
9. 7000 g   **10.** 10 mcg

In metric conversions up the scale, from smaller to larger units of measure, the quantity will get smaller, for example mL to L. The decimal point moves **three places to the left**.

EXAMPLE 1   200 mL = ___.2___ L

You are converting up the scale. Move the decimal point three places left. The quantity becomes smaller 200 mL = 0.2 L (remember the safety feature of adding a zero in front of the decimal).

EXAMPLE 2   500 mcg = ___.5___ mg

Move the decimal point three places to the left. The quantity becomes smaller. 500 mcg = 0.5 mg.

PROBLEM

Convert the following metric measures.

1. 3500 mL = ____3.5____ L
2. 520 mg   = ____.52____ g
3. 1800 mcg = ____1.8____ mg
4. 750 cc   = ____.75____ L
5. 150 mg   = ____.15____ g
6. 250 mcg = ____.25____ mg
7. 1200 mg = ____1.2____ g
8. 600 mL   = ____.6____ L
9. 100 mg   = ____.1____ g
10. 950 mcg = ____.95____ mg

ANSWERS   **1.** 3.5 L   **2.** 0.52 g   **3.** 1.8 mg   **4.** 0.75 L   **5.** 0.15 g   **6.** 0.25 mg   **7.** 1.2 g   **8.** 0.6 L   **9.** 0.1 g
10. 0.95 mg

This concludes your refresher on the metric system. The important points to remember from this chapter are:

■ the meter, liter, and gram are the basic units of metric measures

■ larger and smaller units than the basics are identified by the use of prefixes

■ each prefix changes the value of the basic unit by the same amount

■ converting from one unit to another within the system is accomplished by moving the decimal point

SUMMARY SELF TEST

Metric/SI/International System

1. List the basic units of measure of the metric system and indicate what type of measure they are used for.

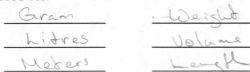

Gram	Weight
Litres	Volume
Meters	Length

2. Which of the following are official metric/SI abbreviations?

   a. L   Litre
   b. g   gram
   c. kL   Kilo litre
   d. mgm   ✗
   e. mg   milligram
   f. kg   kilogram
   g. ml
   h. G   (g)   _____

DIRECTIONS Express the following measures using official metric abbreviations and notation rules.

3. six-hundredths of a milligram   .06 mg
4. three hundred and ten milliliters   310 ml
5. three-tenths of a kilogram   .3 kg
6. four-tenths of a cubic centimeter   .4 cc
7. one and five-tenths grams   1.5 g
8. one-hundredths of a gram   .01 g
9. four thousand milliliters   4000 mL
10. one and two-tenths milligrams   1.2 mg

11. List the four commonly used units of weight and the two of volume, from highest to lowest value.

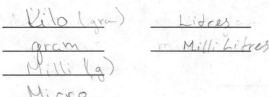

Kilo (gram)	Litres
gram	Milli Litres
Milli (g)	
Micro	

DIRECTIONS Convert the following metric measures.

12. 160 mg   = ___.160___ g

13. 10 kg   = ___10000___ g

14. 1500 µg = ___1,500___ mg   *micro*

15. 750 mg   = ___.75___ g

16. 200 mL   = ___.200___ L

17. 0.3 g   = ___300___ mg

18. 0.05 g   = ___50___ mg

19. 0.15 g   = ___150___ mg

20. 1.2 L   = ___1200___ mL

21. 15 mL   = ___15___ cc

22. 2 mg   = ___2000___ mcg

23. 900 mcg = ___.9___ mg

24. 2.1 L   = ___2100___ mL

25. 475 mL   = ___.475___ L

µ = micro

ANSWERS

1. gram-weight; liter-volume; meter-length **2.** a, b, c, e, f **3.** 0.06 mg **4.** 310 mL **5.** 0.3 kg **6.** 0.4 cc **7.** 1.5 g **8.** 0.01 g
9. 4000 mL **10.** 1.2 mg **11.** kg, g, mg, mcg; L, mL **12.** 0.16 g **13.** 10,000 g **14.** 1.5 mg **15.** 0.75 g **16.** 0.2 L **17.** 300 mg
18. 50 mg **19.** 150 mg **20.** 1200 mL **21.** 15 cc **22.** 2000 mcg **23.** 0.9 mg **24.** 2100 mL **25.** 0.475 L

8

Apothecary and Household Systems

OBJECTIVES
The student will
1. list the symbols, abbreviations, and notation rules for apothecary and household measures
2. convert apothecary and household measures to metric equivalents
3. explain why discrepancies exist in such conversions

INTRODUCTION
The apothecaries' and household are the oldest of the drug measurement systems. Apothecary measures are not frequently used, but you must still be familiar with them and know how to convert them to metric equivalents. Household measures are still in use, especially for patients being cared for at home, and in children's dosages.

• APOTHECARY AND HOUSEHOLD MEASURES •

There are only four apothecary units of measure for which you must memorize the abbreviations and symbols. Take a minute to learn them now and practice printing them before moving ahead in the lesson. The units are as follows:

for weight:	**grain**	**gr**	
for volume:	**minim**	**m**	**min**
	dram	℈	**dr**
	ounce	℥	**oz**

You may initially have difficulty remembering the difference between the symbols for dram and ounce. So let's take a minute to clarify these. **An ounce equals 30 mL,** or a full medication cup in case it's easier for you to relate to that. It is the larger of the two measures and the symbol is likewise larger, having an extra loop on top. In fact it almost looks like oz written carelessly ℥ . **A dram equals 4 mL.** It just covers the bottom of a medication cup and is therefore very small compared with an ounce. Its symbol is also smaller ℈ . It is important not to confuse these symbols because the large difference in measures, 30 mL for ounce is opposed to 4 mL for dram could make errors very serious.

Once again: ounce = ℥ = 30 mL

dram = ℈ = 4 mL

A minim is considered equal in size to a drop, so it is a very small measure.

$$1 \text{ minim} = m \text{ or min} = 1 \text{ drop}$$

Three **household** measures are still in common use:

tablespoon—T or tbs   teaspoon—t or tsp   drop—gtt

Memorize these if you are not already familiar with them. Be careful not to confuse the single letter abbreviations for table and teaspoon. A tablespoon is larger (15 mL) and is printed with a capital T; the teaspoon which is smaller (5 mL), is printed with a small t.

Once again: tablespoon = T or tbs = 15 mL

teaspoon = t or tsp = 5 mL

PROBLEM

Write the symbols and/or abbreviations for the following measures.

1. minim _____ min _____   _____ m _____
2. teaspoon _____ t _____   _____ tsp _____
3. ounce _____ ℥ _____   _____ oz _____
4. grain _____ gr _____   _____
5. dram _____ ℈ _____   _____
6. drop _____ dr _____   _____ gtt _____
7. tablespoon _____ T _____   _____ Tbs _____

ANSWERS   1. min, m   2. t, tsp   3. ℥ , oz   4. gr   5. ℈ , dr   6. gtt   7. T, tbs

• APOTHECARY AND HOUSEHOLD NOTATION RULES •

The best overall description of **apothecary notations** is that they are the exact opposite of metric notations.

RULES: ■ **The symbol is placed in front of the quantity.**

EXAMPLE   gr 7½   gr ¹⁄₁₅₀   (not 7½ gr, ¹⁄₁₅₀ gr)

■ **Fractions are expressed as common fractions in Arabic numerals.**

EXAMPLE   gr ¼   gr ¹⁄₁₅₀

■ **Larger quantities may be written in Roman or Arabic numerals**

EXAMPLE   Roman gr $\overline{VII}$ Arabic gr 7

Need a refresher in Roman numerals? Here's how they are used in medicine (1–10)

$\dot{I}$ $\ddot{II}$ $\dddot{III}$ $\dot{IV}$ $\overline{V}$ $\overline{VI}$ $\overline{VII}$ $\overline{VIII}$ $\dot{IX}$ $\overline{X}$

You should also know 20, $\overline{XX}$ and 30, $\overline{XXX}$ since these are occasionally used. Note that it is the usual practice when writing Roman numerals to **draw a line over the digits, and to dot the numeral 1 (one) each time as a safeguard against errors**. For example, a hastily written 5 ($\overline{V}$) could be mistaken for 2 ($\overline{II}$), but not if each numeral 1 has a dot ($\overset{..}{II}$).

■ **The symbol ss may be used for ½**

EXAMPLE gr $\overset{.}{\overline{Iss}}$ gr $\overline{VIIss}$

If you find memorizing prototypes helpful here are two notations which incorporate all the above rules:

gr 1½   gr $\overline{VIIss}$

There are no standard notation rules for **household measures**, so be prepared to see quite a variety in use, for example 1 T, gtt 2, $\overset{..}{II}$ tsp, etc.

Express the following measures using the abbreviations/symbols and notation rules just discussed.

1. nine and one-half grains .... _gr $\overline{IX}$ ss_   _gr $\overset{.}{\overline{IX\,ss}}$_
2. five minims .... _m $\overline{V}$_
3. one two-hundredths of a grain .... _gr ¹⁄₂₀₀_
4. four ounces .... _℥ $\overline{IV}$_
5. one-sixteenth of a grain .... _gr ¹⁄₁₆_
6. one hundred fiftieth of a grain .... _gr ¹⁄₁₅₀_
7. twenty grains .... _gr $\overline{XX}$_
8. one and one-half grains .... _gr $\overset{.}{\overline{I}}$ ss_   _gr $\overset{.}{\overline{I\,ss}}$_
9. four drams .... _ʒ $\overline{IV}$_
10. three and a half grains .... _ʒ $\overset{...}{\overline{IIIss}}$_
11. two tablespoons .... _T $\overset{..}{II}$_ , T 2, etc
12. six teaspoons .... _t $\overline{VI}$_ , t 6, 6 tsp
13. four drops .... _gtt $\overset{..}{\overline{IV}}$, dr $\overline{IV}$_
14. one-quarter grain .... _gr ¼_
15. one and a half ounces .... _℥ $\overline{Iss}$_ , 1½ oz.

ANSWERS **1.** gr $\overset{.}{\overline{IXss}}$ **2.** m $\overline{V}$, <u>min</u> 5 **3.** gr ½₀₀ **4.** ℥ $\overline{IV}$, oz 4 **5.** gr ¹⁄₁₆ **6.** gr ¹⁄₁₅₀ **7.** gr $\overline{XX}$ **8.** gr $\overline{Iss}$ **9.** ℥ $\overline{IV}$, dr 4 **10.** gr $\overline{IIIss}$ **11.** 2 T, 2 tbs, etc. **12.** 6 t, 6 tsp, etc. **13.** 4 gtt, gtt $\overline{IV}$, etc. **14.** gr ¼ **15.** ℥ $\overline{Iss}$; 1½ oz, etc.

Write the Roman numerals for the following numbers.

1. seven ___ $\overset{..}{VII}$ ___
2. thirty ___ XXX ___

3. four _____

4. one _____

5. nine _____

6. twenty _____

7. two _____

8. five _____

9. eight _____

10. six _____

ANSWERS 1. $\overline{\text{VII}}$ 2. $\overline{\text{XXX}}$ 3. $\overline{\text{IV}}$ 4. $\overline{\text{I}}$ 5. $\overline{\text{IX}}$ 6. $\overline{\text{XX}}$ 7. $\overline{\text{II}}$ 8. $\overline{\text{V}}$ 9. $\overline{\text{VIII}}$ 10. $\overline{\text{VI}}$

• APOTHECARY/HOUSEHOLD/METRIC CONVERSIONS •

Conversion to equivalent measures between systems is necessary when an order is written in one system, but the drug label is stated in another. For example a doctor may order gr ⅙, but the label reads 15 mg. If you do conversions infrequently the safest way to proceed is to refer to a conversion/equivalents table or chart. All hospitals and doctors offices will have one available. Let's begin by looking at a typical conversion/equivalents table. Refer to figure 4, and notice that the equivalents for **liquid** measures are on the left, and for **weight** on the right.

APOTHECARY/HOUSEHOLD/METRIC EQUIVALENTS							
Liquid				**Weight**			
oz	**mL**	**min**	**mL**	**gr**	**mg**	**gr**	**mg**
1	= 30	45	= 3	15	= 1000	1/4	= 15
½	= 15	30	= 2	10	= 600	1/6	= 10
		15	= 1	7½	= 500	1/8	= 8
dr	**mL**	12	= 0.75	5	= 300	1/10	= 6
2½	= 10	10	= 0.6	4	= 250	1/15	= 4
2	= 8	8	= 0.5	3	= 200	1/20	= 3
1¼	= 5	5	= 0.3	2½	= 150	1/30	= 2
1	= 4	4	= 0.25	2	= 120	1/40	= 1.5
1 min =	1 gtt	3	= 0.2	1½	= 100	1/60	= 1
1 T	= 15 mL	1½	= 0.1	1	= 60	1/100	= 0.6
1 t	= 5 mL	1	= 0.06	3/4	= 45	1/120	= 0.5
		¾	= 0.05	1/2	= 30	1/150	= 0.4
		½	= 0.03	1/3	= 20	1/200	= 0.3
						1/250	= 0.25

Figure 4

The numbers on this conversion table, as on most conversion tables, are small and close together. This contributes to the most common error in the use of conversion tables, which is to misread from one column to another. For example, if you are converting gr ⅛ to mg, it is not impossible to incorrectly read one line above the correct equivalent, 10 mg, or one line below, 6 mg. To eliminate this possibility **always use a guide to read from one column to the other**. Use any straight edge available and you will see immediately that gr ⅛ is equivalent to 8 mg. Very simple, very safe.

PROBLEM

Use the conversion table in figure 4 to determine the following equivalent measures.

1. gr ¼ = ___15___ mg

2. 30 mL = oz ___1___

3. 100 mg = gr ___1 ½___

4. gr ⅙ = ___10___ mg

5. 60 mg = gr ___1___

6. 4 mL = dr ___1___

7. gr 7½ = ___500___ mg

8. oz ½ = ___15___ mL

9. 300 mg = gr ___5___

10. 15 mg = gr ___¼___

11. gr ¹/₁₀₀ = ___.6___ mg

12. 0.4 mg = gr ___¹/₁₅₀___

13. 2 min = ___20___ gtt

14. 30 mg = gr ___½___

15. 10 mL = ___2___ t

16. 2 T = ___30___ mL

ANSWERS   **1.** 15 mg   **2.** 1 oz   **3.** gr 1½   **4.** 10 mg   **5.** gr 1   **6.** dr 1   **7.** 500 mg   **8.** 15 mL   **9.** gr 5   **10.** gr ¼
11. 0.6 mg   **12.** gr ¹/₁₅₀   **13.** 2 gtt   **14.** gr ½   **15.** 2 t   **16.** 30 mL

• DISCREPANCIES IN EQUIVALENTS •

There is an inconsistency in conversions that you need to be aware of. The conversion table you just used is in fact a table of **equivalent**, not **exact** measures. To illustrate this read the dosage strengths which are circled on the labels in figures 5 and 6.

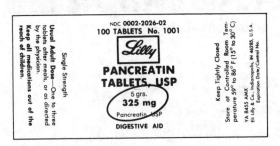

Figure 5

Figure 6

As you can see the label in figure 5 indicates that 5 gr equals 325 mg, while the label in figure 10 states that 300 mg equals 5 gr. Which is correct? In fact they both are, and you need to understand why.

Your table of equivalents tells you that gr 1 equals 60 mg. In actual fact it equals approximately 64 mg. However, the tendency is to round off the numbers, so you are more likely to see 60 mg than 64 mg. But you may well see both. You will also see gr ½ listed as 30 mg, and 32 mg. And you have just discovered that gr 5 is equivalent to 300 mg, and 325 mg. You may also see it recorded as 324 mg.

The point being reinforced here is that conversions are **equivalent** not **equal** measures. The discrepancy results from the fact that the apothecaries' system is so inaccurate. The original gr was defined as the weight of a grain of wheat, which will give you some idea what an obsolete system of measure the apothecaries' is. So, don't be surprised when you see small discrepancies, they do exist. The important thing is that you **question all inconsistencies you are unfamiliar with**, and keep in mind that the **smaller the dosage the more significant the discrepancy will be**. For example, the difference between 300 and 325 mg may be slight in terms of drug action; the difference between 0.3 and 0.4 mg is enormous, since the drug potency is obviously so much greater. **Never guess at equivalents, take the time to be absolutely certain.**

• CALCULATING EQUIVALENTS MATHEMATICALLY •

Some equivalents are so common that you should memorize them. For example 60 mg = gr 1. If you know this equivalent it is then very easy to mentally calculate close multiples and fractions.

EXAMPLE
$$
\begin{aligned}
60 \text{ mg} &= \text{gr } 1 \\
120 \text{ mg} &= \text{gr } 2 \\
30 \text{ mg} &= \text{gr } \tfrac{1}{2} \\
15 \text{ mg} &= \text{gr } \tfrac{1}{4}
\end{aligned}
$$

Here are several equivalents which you could memorize, because they are used fairly often.

$$
\begin{aligned}
\text{gr } 1 &= 60 \text{ mg} \\
\text{gr } 5 &= 300 \text{ mg} \\
\text{gr } 15 &= 1000 \text{ mg (1g)} \\
\text{gr } \tfrac{1}{150} &= 0.4 \text{ mg} \\
1 \text{ oz} &= 30 \text{ mL} \\
1 \text{ dr} &= 4 \text{ mL} \\
1 \text{ T} &= 15 \text{ mL} \\
1 \text{ t} &= 5 \text{ mL}
\end{aligned}
$$

PROBLEM

Use the equivalents just discussed to convert the following measures.

1. gr ¾   = ____45____ mg
2. gr ¼   = ____15____ mg
3. ½ oz   = ____15____ mL
4. gr 15   = ____1000____ mg
5. 8 mL   = dr ____2____
6. 300 mg   = gr ____5____
7. gr ⅟₁₀₀   = ____.6____ mg
8. 10 mL   = ____2____ t
9. dr i̇   = ____4____ mL
10. 2 T   = ____30____ mL

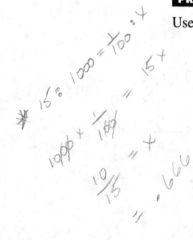

You can also calculate equivalents mathematically using ratio and proportion (see Chapter 5). All you will need to know is one equivalent.

EXAMPLE 1 You must convert gr ⅙ to mg. You know that gr 1 = 60 mg. This is the complete or known ratio, so always write it first.

gr 1 : 60 mg

Then add the incomplete ratio, making sure it is written in the same sequence of measurement units, gr : mg

gr 1 : 60 **mg** = **gr** ⅙ : X **mg**
60 × ⅙ = X = 10 mg

EXAMPLE 2 The drug label reads 0.4 mg. A dosage of gr ¹⁄₁₅₀ is ordered. Are these the same dosage?

gr 1 : 60 mg = gr ¹⁄₁₅₀ : X mg
60 x ¹⁄₁₅₀ = X = 0.4 mg

Answer: gr ¹⁄₁₅₀ = 0.4 mg   These dosages are the same

PROBLEM

Use ratio and proportion to determine metric equivalents for the following apothecary measures.

1. gr ¼ = _____15_____ mg
2. gr ¹⁄₂₀₀ = _____.3_____ mg

This concludes your introduction to the apothecaries' and household systems of measure. The important points to remember from this chapter are:

- the four apothecary measures sometimes used are the grain, minim, dram, and ounce

- a minim is equal in size to a drop

- the three household measures still in use today are the tablespoon, teaspoon, and drop

- there are no standard notation rules for household measures

- the symbol is placed in front of the number in apothecary notations

- refer to a conversion table to determine metric, apothecary, and household equivalents

- conversions between metric and apothecary/household measures are equivalent not equal measures

- calculating equivalents between two systems is easiest using the method of ratio and proportion

■ always write the complete or known ratio first then the incomplete ratio using the same sequence of measurement units

Apothecary/Household Systems

DIRECTIONS What unit of measure do the following symbols/abbreviations identify?

1. ʒ ___dram___
2. oz ___ounce___
3. m ___minim___
4. dr ___dram___
5. gtt ___drop___
6. ℥ ___ounce___
7. t ___teaspoon___
8. min ___minim___
9. T ___tablespoon___
10. gr ___grain___
11. tsp ___teaspoon___
12. tbs ___tablespoon___

DIRECTIONS Write the dosages identified by the following notations.

13. ʒ $\overline{IV}$ ___4 drams___
14. $\overline{II}$ T ___2 Teaspoons___
15. gr $\overline{IIIss}$ ___3 ½ grains___
16. ℥ $\overline{I}$ ___1 ounce___
17. $\overline{II}$ tsp ___2 tspoons___
18. 3 gtt ___3 drops___
19. gr $\overline{VIIss}$ ___7 ½ grains___
20. oz 3 ___℥ $\overline{III}$ 3 ounces___
21. dr $\overline{I}$ ___One dram___
22. gr ¹/₁₀₀ ___one one hundredth grain___

DIRECTIONS Convert the following to the equivalent measures specified. You may use the equivalents you have memorized, the equivalents table on page 66 or ratio and proportion for this section.

23. 3 T = ___45___ mL
24. gr ½ = ___30___ mg
25. 1 mL = min ___15___
26. 15 mL = ___1___ tbs

27. ℥ ÏÏ   = _____8_____ mL

28. gr Ï   = _____60_____ mg

29. gr 5   = _____300_____ mg

30. 1 g   = gr _____ ✳ ,

31. 4 tsp   = _____20_____ mL

32. 500 mg = gr ____7.5_____

33. gr ½   = _____30_____ mg

34. gr ¹⁄₁₅₀ = _____.4_____ mg ✳

.5oz 35. ℥ s̄s   = _____15_____ mL

36. 1 min   = _____1_____ gtt

37. 1 t   = _____15_____ mL

38. 1 oz   = _____30_____ mL

39. 1 tbs   = _____15_____ mL

40. gr ¼   = _____15_____ mg

Handwritten work (right margin):
$$\frac{3:200}{4} = \frac{\frac{1}{150}:x}{}$$
$$200 \times \frac{\frac{1}{150}}{3} = \frac{\frac{1}{3}}{}$$
$$\frac{4}{3} \times \frac{1}{3}$$
$$\frac{4}{9}$$
$$x = .4$$

ANSWERS

1. dram 2. ounce 3. minim 4. dram 5. drop 6. ounce 7. teaspoon 8. minim 9. tablespoon 10. grain 11. teaspoon
12. tablespoon 13. 4 drams 14. 2 tablespoons 15. 3½ grains 16. 1 ounce 17. 2 teaspoons 18. 3 drops 19. 7½ grains
20. 3 ounces 21. 1 dram 22. ¹⁄₁₀₀ grain 23. 45 mL 24. 30 mg 25. min 15 26. 1 tbs 27. 8 mL 28. 60 mg 29. 300 mg
30. gr 15 31. 20 mL 32. gr 7½ 33. 30 mg 34. 0.4 mg 35. 15 mL 36. 1 gtt 37. 5 mL 38. 30 mL 39. 15 mL
40. 15 mg

SECTION
THREE

Reading Medication Labels and Syringe Calibrations

9
Reading Oral Medication Labels

OBJECTIVES
The student will
1. identify scored tablets, unscored tablets, and capsules
2. read drug labels to identify trade and generic names
3. identify dosage strengths and calculate simple dosages
4. measure oral solutions using a medicine cup and calibrated dropper

INTRODUCTION
Medication labels contain a variety of information, which ranges from simple to complex. In this chapter you will be introduced to labels of oral medications which are generally the least complicated. With this instruction you will be able to locate drugs and calculate simple dosages without confusion, as well as understand the more complicated labels presented in later chapters. We will begin with labels for solid drug preparations. These include tablets; scored tablets (which contain an indented marking to make breakage for partial dosages possible); enteric coated tablets (which delay absorption until the drug reaches the small intestine); and capsules (powdered or oily drugs in a gelatin cover). See illustrations in figure 7.

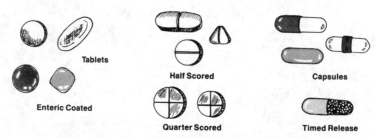

Figure 7

• READING TABLET AND CAPSULE LABELS •

The most common type of label currently in use is the **unit dosage label**, in which a single tablet or capsule is packaged separately.

EXAMPLE 1   Look at the Lanoxin label in figure 8

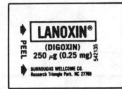

Figure 8

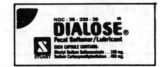

Figure 9

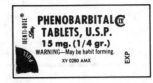

Figure 10

The first thing to notice is that this drug has two names. The first, Lanoxin, is its **trade name**, which is identified by the ® registration symbol. Trade names are usually capitalized and printed first on the label. The name in smaller print, digoxin, is the **generic or official name** of the drug. Each drug has only one official name, but may have several trade names, each for the exclusive use of the company which manufactures it. It is important to remember, however, that the label does contain **both** names, because drugs may be ordered by either name depending on hospital policy or physician preference. You will frequently need to cross check names for accurate drug identification.

Next on the label is the **dosage strength**, 250 mcg (written with its SI symbol, μg) or 0.25 mg. The dosage is often representative of the **average dosage strength, the dosage given to the average patient at one time**. This label also identifies the manufacturer of this drug, Burroughs Wellcome Co.

EXAMPLE 2   The Dialose® label in figure 9 lists the names and amounts of two generic drugs: dioctyl sodium sulfosuccinate 100 mg, and sodium carboxymethylcellulose 400 mg. It is not uncommon for tablets or capsules to contain more than one drug, and when this is the case dosages are usually ordered by numbers of tablets or capsules to be administered, rather than by drug strength. Notice that no dosage strength is given for Dialose®, and for combination drugs this is frequently the case.

EXAMPLE 3   The label in figure 10 bears only one name, phenobarbital, which is actually the generic name of the drug. This is common with drugs which have been in use for many years. The official (generic) name was so well established that drug manufacturers did not try to promote their own trade names. Also notice that immediately after the drug name are the initials **U.S.P.** This is the abbreviation for **United States Pharmacopeia**, one of the two official national listings of drugs. The other is the **National Formulary, N.F.** You will see U.S.P. and N.F. on drug labels, and must not confuse this with other initials which identify additional drugs in a preparation.

Next, notice that this label gives the dosage strength of phenobarbital in both metric and apothecaries' units of measure, 15 mg and gr ¼. Finally, on the right of the label, printed sideways, are the letters "EXP". This represents "expiration"; the last date when the drug should be used. Make a habit of checking the expiration dates on labels.

PROBLEM

Refer to the label in figure 11 and answer the following questions about this drug.

  1. What is the generic name? _____

  2. What is the trade name? _____

3. What is the dosage strength? _____

4. What is the expiration date? _____

ANSWERS 1. propantheline bromide   2. Pro-Banthine®   3. 15 mg   4. 6-6-98

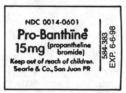
Figure 11

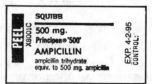
Figure 12

PROBLEM

Refer to the label in figure 12 and answer the following questions about this drug.

1. What is the generic name? _____

2. What is the trade name? _____

3. What is the dosage strength? _____

4. What is the expiration date? _____

ANSWERS 1. ampicillin trihydate   2. Principen®   3. 500 mg (If you said the dosage strength was 500 you were only half right. Dosage strengths must always be expressed with a unit of measure, in this case mg, 500 mg)
4. expires 4-2-95

While most drugs are available in the unit dosage format, you may occasionally see packages or bottles containing multiple capsules or tablets. The labels are slightly larger, and contain more information. Refer to the Vistaril label in figure 13.

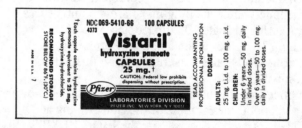
Figure 13

Notice that this label contains dosage information on the right side, and storage information on the left, but basically it is the same as the smaller unit dosage labels you are now familiar with. There is only one area you should be aware of that might cause confusion. Notice the number 100 (capsules) in the upper right hand corner. This indicates that the **total number** of capsules in the bottle is 100. Be careful not to confuse this number with the dosage strength. **The dosage strength always has a unit of measure beside it**, in this case mg, 25 mg.

• CALCULATING SIMPLE DOSAGES •

When the time comes for you to administer medications you will have to read a medication record or Kardex to prepare the dosage. This will tell you the name and amount of drug to be given, but **it will not tell you how many tablets or capsules contain this dosage**. This you must calculate yourself. However, this is not difficult. Most tablets/capsules are prepared in average dosage strengths, and most orders will involve giving one to three tablets. **Learn to question orders for more than three tablets.** Although a few drugs require multiple tablets, most do not, and an unusual number could be a warning of an error in prescribing, transcribing, or your calculations. **Regardless of the source of an error, if you give a wrong dosage you are legally responsible for it.** Occasionally a dosage will require half of a tablet but this would only be the case if the tablet were scored and could be accurately broken in half. (Refer to figure 7 for illustrations of score marks). Let's look at some sample orders and do some actual dosage calculations. Assume that both tablets in our problems are scored.

Figure 14

Figure 15

PROBLEM

Refer to the Kenacort® label in figure 14 and answer the following questions.

1. What is the dosage strength? _____

2. If you have an order for 4 mg give _____

3. If you have an order for 6 mg give _____

4. If 12 mg are ordered give _____

ANSWERS   **1.** 4 mg   **2.** 1 tab   **3.** 1½ tab   **4.** 3 tabs

---

PROBLEM

Refer to the Hexadrol® label in figure 15 and answer the following questions.

1. What is the dosage strength? _____

2. If 0.25 mg are ordered give _____

3. If 1 mg is ordered give _____

4. If 0.5 mg are ordered give _____

ANSWERS   **1.** 0.5 mg   **2.** ½ tab   **3.** 2 tab   **4.** 1 tab

Dosages will frequently have to be converted from one metric unit of measure to another, for example from mg to mcg, or g to mg.

PROBLEM

Calculate the following dosages using the Kenacort® and Hexadrol® labels in figures 14 and 15

1. Kenacort® 2000 mcg are ordered. Give _____ ½ _____ tab
2. Hexadrol® 250 mcg are ordered. Give _____ ½ _____ tab
3. Hexadrol® 500 mcg are ordered. Give _____ 1 _____ tab

ANSWERS 1. ½ tab. The strength is 4 mg, or 4000 mcg   2. ½ tab. The strength is 0.5 mg or 500 mcg
3. 1 tab. 0.5 mg equals 500 mcg

PROBLEM

Locate the appropriate labels below for the following drug orders and indicate the number of tablets/capsules which will be required to administer the dosages ordered. Assume that all tablets are scored. Notice that both generic and trade names are used for the orders.

1. isosorbide dinitrate 80 mg _____ 2 _____ tab
2. sulfasalazine 0.5 g _____ 1 _____ tab
3. sulfasalazine 1 g _____ 2 _____ tab
4. hydrochlorothiazide 25 mg _____ ½ _____ tab
5. chlordiazepoxide HCl 50 mg _____ 2 _____ cap
6. Stelazine® 7.5 mg _____ 1 ½ _____ tab
7. Minipress® 2 mg _____ 1 _____ cap
8. phenytoin Na 90 mg _____ 3 _____ cap
9. diphenhydramine HCl 100 mg _____ 2 _____ cap
10. allopurinal 450 mg _____ 1 ½ _____ tab

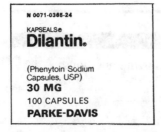

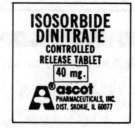

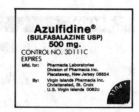

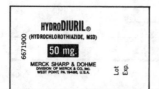

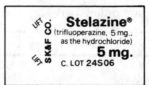

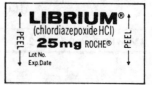

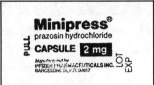
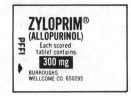

ANSWERS **1.** 2 tab **2.** 1 tab **3.** 2 tab **4.** ½ tab **5.** 2 cap **6.** 1½ tab **7.** 1 cap **8.** 3 cap **9.** 2 cap
10. 1½ tab

• READING ORAL SOLUTION LABELS •

You have just learned that in solid drug preparations, for example tablets, each tablet contained a certain weight of drug, for example 250 mg. In liquid preparations the weight of the drug is contained in a certain **volume of solution**, most frequently mL or cc's. Let's compare a solid and liquid drug preparation to illustrate the difference.

EXAMPLE 1   **Solid:** 250 mg in **1 tablet**   **Liquid:** 250 mg in **5 mL**

EXAMPLE 2   **Solid:** 100 mg in **1 capsule**   **Liquid:** 100 mg in **10 mL**

    Solution strength can also be expressed in ounces, drams, teaspoons or tablespoons, but these measures are less common. Let's look at some solution labels so that you can become familiar with them.

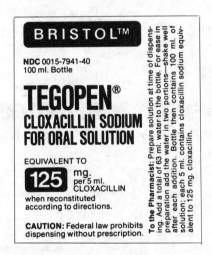

Figure 16

    Refer to the Tegopen® label in figure 16. The information it contains will be familiar. Tegopen® is the trade name, cloxacillin sodium is the generic or official name. The **dosage strength is 125 mg per 5 mL**, and the total volume of the bottle is 100 mL.

    As with solid drugs the medication record will tell you the dosage of the drug to be administered, but rarely will it specify the volume which contains this dosage.

PROBLEM

Refer to the cloxacillin label in figure 16 again, and calculate the following dosages.

1. The order is for 125 mg. Give _____5_____
2. The order is for 0.25 g. Give _____10_____

ANSWERS   **1.** 5 mL   **2.** 10 mL

(handwritten in left margin:)
$.25 g = 250 mg$
$125 = 5$
$250 = x$
$x = 10$

If you did not express your answers as mL they are incorrect. Numbers have no meaning unless they are expressed with a unit of measure, in this case mL.

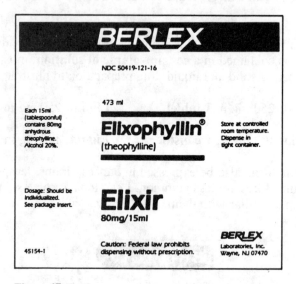

Figure 17

PROBLEM

Refer to the Elixophyllin® label in figure 17, and calculate the following dosages.

1. The order is for 160 mg. Give _____30 ml_____
2. The order is for 40 mg. Give _____7.5 ml_____
3. 80 mg has been ordered. Give _____15 ml_____

(handwritten in left margin:)
$mg\ 80 = 15\ ml$
$160 = 30$
$40 = 7.5$

ANSWERS   **1.** 30 mL   **2.** 7.5 mL   **3.** 15 mL   Your answers are incorrect unless they include mL as the unit of measure.

PROBLEM

Refer to the appropriate label in figures 18 and 19 to calculate the following oral solution dosages.

1. hetacillin 225 mg _____10 ml_____
2. digoxin 50 mcg _____1_____
3. Lanoxin® 0.1 mg _____

(handwritten in left margin:)
112.5
225.0

    4. Versapen® 112.5 mg ___*5 ml*___

    5. digoxin 75 mcg ___*1.5 cc*___

ANSWERS   **1.** 10 mL   **2.** 1 cc   **3.** 2 cc   **4.** 5 mL   **5.** 1.5 cc

---

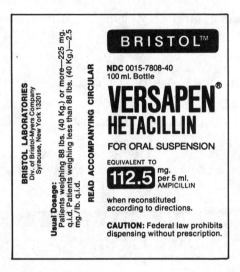

Figure 18

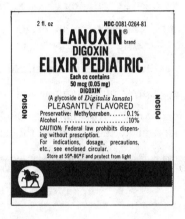

Figure 19

• MEASUREMENT OF ORAL SOLUTIONS •

Oral solutions can be measured using a calibrated medicine cup such as the one shown in figure 20. Notice that it contains calibrations in mL (cc), tbs, tsp, dr, and oz. To pour accurately hold the cup at eye level, then line up the measure you need and pour. Volumes of less than 5 mL are frequently measured using a hypodermic syringe (with the needle removed), or an oral syringe with the same calibrations, but a different shaped hub. Syringe measurements will be covered in detail in the next chapter.

    Oral solutions may also be ordered as drops (gtt), and when this is the case the dropper is usually attached to the bottle stopper. It is also common for medicine droppers to be calibrated, for example in mL as in figure 21 or by actual dosage, 125 mg, 250 mg, etc.

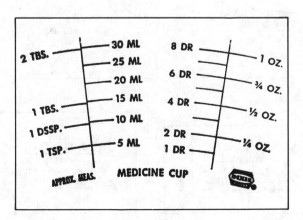

Figure 20

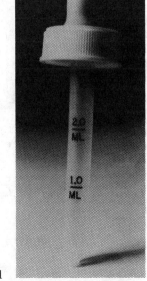

Figure 21

This concludes the chapter on reading oral medication labels. The following are important points to remember:

- most labels contain both generic and trade names

- dosages are clearly printed on the label, except for preparations containing multiple drugs which are sold under trade names only. Example: Dialose®

- do not confuse the single letter designations on labels with the U.S.P. or N.F. which identifies national drug listings

- check drug expiration dates before use

- most dosages of oral medications will involve giving 1–3 tablets/capsules. Question dosages which appear too large

- oral solution dosages are measured in cc's, oz, tsp, tbs, or gtt

- for accurate measurement oral solutions are poured at eye level

- small volumes of solutions may be measured (and administered) with an oral or hypodermic syringe (without the needle)

SUMMARY SELF TEST

Reading Oral Medication Labels

DIRECTIONS Locate the appropriate label for each of the following drug orders, and indicate the number of tablets/capsules or mL/cc which will be required to administer them.

PART I

1. acetaminophen 650 mg ___2 tab___
2. Aldactone® 75 mg ___3 tab___
3. meclizine HCl 50 mg ___2 tab___
4. Reglan® 15 mg ___1.5 tab___
5. propranolol HCl 30 mg ___1.5 tab___
6. metroprolol tartrate 0.15 g ___1.5 tab___

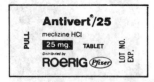
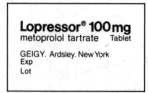
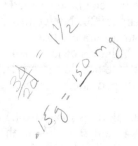
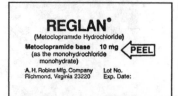
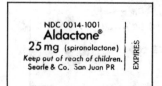
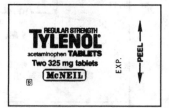
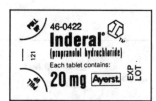

PART II

7. nifedipine 10 mg _____ 1 cap

8. furosemide 10 mg _____ 2 tab

9. Lasix® 30 mg _____ 1.5 tab

10. Tagamet® 0.3 g _____ 3 tab

11. clonidine HCl 200 mcg _____ 2 tab

12. dexamethasone 3 mg _____ 1.5 tab

13. Tenormin® 0.15 g _____ 1.5 tab

14. terbutaline 2.5 mg _____ 2 tab

15. Procan® 0.75 g _____ 1 tab

16. Synthroid® 225 mcg _____ 1.5 tab

N 0054-8176 **2 mg**
DEXAMETHASONE
Tablet USP, 2 mg
LOT   EXP.
Roxane Laboratories

LIFT SK&F LAB CO. Carolina, P.R. LIFT **Tagamet®**
(cimetidine)
300mg. Tablet
C. LOT
EXPIRES

Catapres®.1
(clonidine HCl USP) 0.1 mg
LOT
EXP.
Boehringer Ingelheim Ltd.
Ridgefield, CT 06877
PEEL TO OPEN

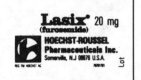

Lasix® 20 mg
(furosemide)
HOECHST-ROUSSEL
Pharmaceuticals Inc.
Somerville, N.J. 08876 U.S.A.
REG TM HOECHST AG
Lot

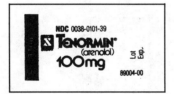

NDC 0038-0101-39
TENORMIN®
(atenolol)
100mg
Lot
Exp.
89004-00

Procardia®
nifedipine
CAPSULE **10mg**
Pfizer Inc., New York, N.Y. 10017

PULL
Synthroid® 150 mcg
(Levothyroxine Sodium
Tablets, USP)
Travenol Laboratories, Inc.
LOT
EXP

Brethine® 5mg
terbutaline sulfate USP Tablet
GEIGY Ardsley, New York
Exp.
Lot   670204

Procan® SR 750 mg
(Procainamide HCl Tablets)
Sustained Release
PARKE-DAVIS
Div of Warner-Lambert Co Lot
Morris Plains, NJ 07950 Exp.
PULL

PART III

17. codeine gr 2 _____ *2 tabs*

18. codeine 30 mg _____ *1/2 tab*

19. rauwolfia 100 mg _____ *2 tabs*

20. Thyroid® gr 1 _____ *2 tab*

✳ **21.** acetaminophen syrup 180 mg _____

22. Dynapen® susp. 62.5 mg _____ *5 ml*

23. dicloxacillin Na susp. 125 mg _____ *10 ml*

24. Colace® syrup 10 mg _____ *2.5 ml*

✳ **25.** Polymox® susp. 75 mg _____ *1.5 ml*

✳ **26.** amoxicillin susp. 0.2 g _____

27. ampicillin susp. 0.5 g _____ *10 ml*

28. Principen® susp. 375 mg _____

29. Elixir Benadryl® 12.5 mg _____

30. diphenhydramine HCl elixir 25 mg _____

$$\frac{62.5}{125.0} \bigg/ 2$$

$$0.50\ mg = \frac{0.25 = .05\ g}{2\sqrt{05.0}}$$

$$\frac{375}{250} :: x :: .5 \\ 50\%\ 1$$

ANSWERS

1. 2 tab **2.** 3 tab **3.** 2 tab **4.** 1½ tab **5.** 1½ tab **6.** 1½ tab **7.** 1 cap **8.** ½ tab **9.** 1½ tab **10.** 1 tab **11.** 2 tab **12.** 1½ tab **13.** 1½ tab **14.** ½ tab **15.** 1 tab **16.** 1½ tab **17.** 2 tab **18.** ½ tab **19.** 2 tab **20.** 2 tab **21.** 7.5 mL **22.** 5 mL **23.** 10 mL **24.** 2.5 mL **25.** 1.5 mL **26.** 4 mL **27.** 10 mL **28.** 7.5 mL **29.** 5 mL **30.** 10 mL

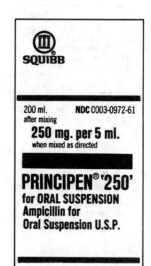

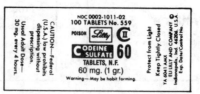

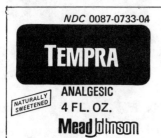

NDC 0087-0733-04

TEMPRA

NATURALLY SWEETENED

ANALGESIC
4 FL. OZ.

Mead Johnson

Each teaspoonful (5 ml.) of TEMPRA® Syrup contains 120 mg. (2 grains) of acetaminophen in 10% alcohol with a delicious, naturally-sweetened cherry flavor. (No artificial sweeteners used.)

Your physician is the best source of counsel and guidance when pain or fever is present.

TEMPRA Syrup is also available in bottles of 16 fl. oz. TEMPRA cherry-flavored drops for infants are available in bottles of ½ fl. oz. (15 ml.) for use as directed by your physician.

Made in U.S.A.   © M. J. & Co.

MEAD JOHNSON NUTRITIONAL DIVISION
Mead Johnson & Company
Evansville, Indiana 47721 U.S.A.

P 7821-02

BRISTOL™

NDC 0015-7277-16
15 ml. Bottle

POLYMOX®
AMOXICILLIN FOR ORAL SUSPENSION
PEDIATRIC DROPS
EQUIVALENT TO
50 mg. per ml. AMOXICILLIN
when reconstituted according to directions.

CAUTION: Federal law prohibits dispensing without prescription.

To the Pharmacist: Prepare suspension at time of dispensing. Add 9 ml. water to the bottle and shake well. This provides 15 ml. of suspension. When prepared as directed, each ml. contains amoxicillin trihydrate equivalent to 50 mg. amoxicillin. Dropper delivers 25 mg. (½ full), and 50 mg. (full).
LIFT HERE

NDC 0087-0720-01

SYRUP

COLACE®
DIOCTYL SODIUM SULFOSUCCINATE
STOOL SOFTENER

8 FL. OZ. (½ PT.)

Mead Johnson

The effect of COLACE on the stools may not be apparent until 1 to 3 days after first oral dose.

Each teaspoon (5 ml.) contains 20 mg. dioctyl sodium sulfosuccinate; each tablespoon (15 ml.) contains 60 mg. Contains not more than 1% alcohol.

Made in U.S.A.   © M.J. & Co.

MEAD JOHNSON PHARMACEUTICAL DIVISION
Mead Johnson & Company
Evansville, Indiana 47721 U.S.A.

P 7169-04

BRISTOL LABORATORIES

Div of Bristol-Myers Company, Syracuse, New York 13201

Usual Dosage: Children weighing less than 40 Kg (88 lbs)—12.5 mg Kg day in equally-divided doses q 6h Adults and children weighing 40 Kg (88 lbs) or more—125 mg q 6h

READ ACCOMPANYING CIRCULAR

To the Pharmacist: Prepare suspension at time of dispensing. 1. Shake container to loosen powder. 2. Measure 57 ml of water for reconstitution. 3. Add approximately one-half the water, **immediately shake vigorously**. 4. Add remaining water and shake vigorously. Bottle then contains 100 ml of suspension. **Note:** This bottle is oversized to **provide greater shake space for ease in reconstitution.** Each 5 ml contains dicloxacillin sodium monohydrate equivalent to 62.5 mg dicloxacillin

*Normal handling may lead to lumps which are not dispersed with continued shaking

© 1977 Bristol Laboratories

BRISTOL®   NDC 0015-7856-40
100 ml BOTTLE

LIFT HERE

Dynapen®
DICLOXACILLIN SODIUM FOR ORAL SUSPENSION
EQUIVALENT TO

62.5 mg per 5 ml

DICLOXACILLIN
when reconstituted according to directions.

CAUTION: Federal law prohibits dispensing without prescription.

ELIXIR

Benadryl

(Diphenhydramine Hydrochloride Elixir)

Caution—Federal law prohibits dispensing without prescription.

4 FLUIDOUNCES
PARKE-DAVIS

Contains—12.5 mg diphenhydramine hydrochloride in each 5 ml; Alcohol, 14%.

Dose—Adults, 2 to 4 teaspoonfuls; children over 20 lb, 1 to 2 teaspoonfuls; infants and children under 20 lb, 1/2 to 1 teaspoonful; three or four times daily.

See package insert.

Keep this and all drugs out of the reach of children.

Store below 86° F (30° C).

Exp date and lot

Stock 9-220-509
Parke, Davis & Co
Detroit, Mi 48232 USA

10
Hypodermic Syringe Measurement

OBJECTIVES
The student will measure parenteral solutions using
1. a standard 3 cc syringe
2. a tuberculin syringe
3. Tubex® and Carpuject® cartridges
4. 5, 6, 10 and 12 cc syringes
5. a 20 cc syringe

INTRODUCTION
A variety of hypodermic syringes are in common use. They have different capacities (3 cc, 6 cc, 20 cc, etc.) and different calibrations. All are calibrated in cc's, but the smaller capacity syringes are further divided into tenths, or two-tenths, or hundredths of a cc. The objective of this chapter is to teach you how to read syringe calibrations, so that you will be comfortable with **any** type of syringe you may encounter.

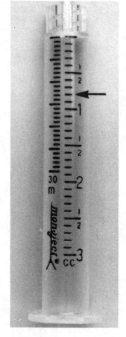

Figure 22

• STANDARD 3 cc SYRINGE •

The most commonly used hypodermic syringe is the 3 cc size illustrated in figure 22. Look at the calibrations on the right side, for metric (cc) measures. The first thing to notice about any syringe is exactly how many calibrations there are in each 1 cc. On this 3 cc syringe there are ten calibrations in each cc, which indicates that the syringe is calibrated in tenths. Larger calibrations identify the 0, ½ (0.5), and full cc measures. The shorter calibrations between these identify the tenths. For example the arrow in figure 22 identifies 0.8 cc.

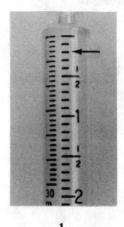

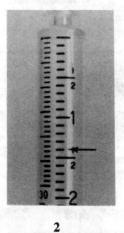

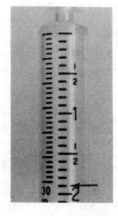

| 1 | 2 | 3 |

Figure 23

PROBLEM

Use decimal numbers for example 2.2 cc, to identify the measurements indicated by the arrows on the standard 3 cc syringes in figure 23.

1. _____   **2.** _____   **3.** _____

ANSWERS   **1.** 0.2 cc   **2.** 1.4 cc   **3.** 1.9 cc

Did you have difficulty with 0.2 cc calibration in problem 1? Remember that the first long calibration on all syringes is zero. It is slightly longer than the 0.1 cc and subsequent one tenth calibrations. Be careful not to mistakenly count it as 0.1 cc.

You have just been looking at photos of syringe barrels only. Next look at the assembled syringes in figure 24. Notice that the black suction tip of the plunger has two widened areas in contact with the barrel, which look like two distinct rings. Calibrations are read from the front, or top ring. Do not become confused by the second, bottom ring, or by the raised middle section of the suction tip.

PROBLEM

What dosages are measured by the three assembled syringes in figure 24?

1. _____   **2.** _____   **3.** _____

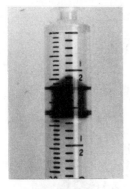 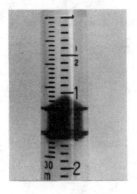 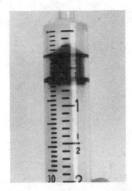

Figure 24

ANSWERS   **1.** 0.7 cc   **2.** 1.2 cc   **3.** 0.3 cc

Refer back to figure 22 and look at the small calibrations on the left of the barrel. This is the minim (m) scale of the apothecaries' system. These calibrations measure a total of 30 m, with larger calibrations identifying each five m increment, for example 5, 10, etc. Only the 30 m calibration is numbered. This scale is not frequently used, but you should be aware that the syringe contains it.

Draw an arrow or shade in the following syringe barrels to indicate the required dosages. Have your instructor double check your accuracy.

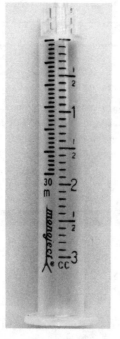

1. 1.3 cc

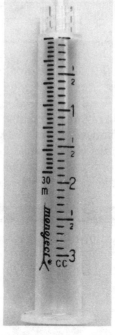

2. 2.4 cc

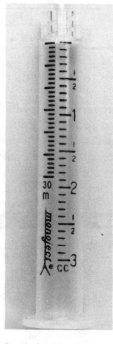

3. 0.9 cc

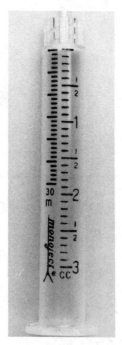

4. 2.5 cc

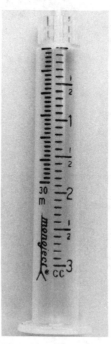

5. 1.7 cc

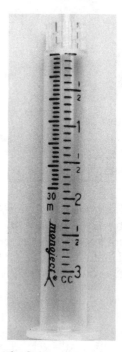

6. 2.1 cc

Identify the dosages measured on the following 3 cc syringes.

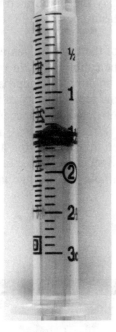

1. _____

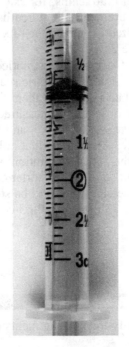

2. _____

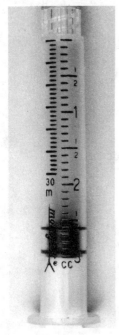

3. _____

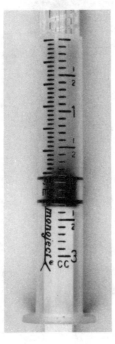

4. _____

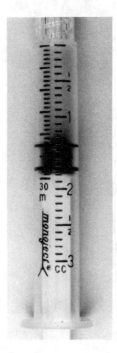

5. _____

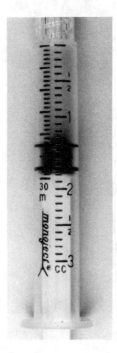

6. _____

ANSWERS   **1.** 1.5 cc   **2.** 2.3 cc   **3.** 0.8 cc   **4.** 2.6 cc   **5.** 1.9 cc   **6.** 1.4 cc

• TUBERCULIN SYRINGE •

When dosages of small volumes are necessary they are measured in hundredths, rather than tenths, for example 0.27 cc, and 0.64 cc. Pediatric dosages usually require measurement in hundredths, as does heparin. A special 1 cc syringe calibrated in hundredths, called the tuberculin (TB), is used for these measurements. Refer to figure 25.

Once again first notice the 30 minim scale on the left of the barrel. Then take a close look at the metric scale on the right. As you can see the calibrations are very small and close together. This mandates particular care and an unhurried approach when dosages are measured using this syringe. Notice that the total capacity of the syringe is 1.00 (1 cc), and that larger calibrations identify zero, and each successive .05 cc. Also notice that only alternate tenths are numbered: .20, .40, .60 etc., and that the actual calibration which identifies these falls between the 2 and 0, the 4 and 0, and so on. The shorter calibrations measure hundredths. Spend some time examining the calibrations to be sure you understand them. For example, the syringe in figure 25 measures 0.63 cc.

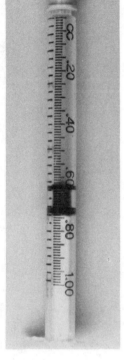

Figure 25

PROBLEM

Identify the measurements on the tuberculin syringes below.

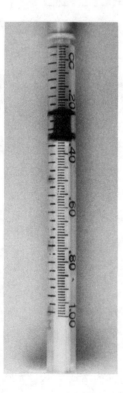 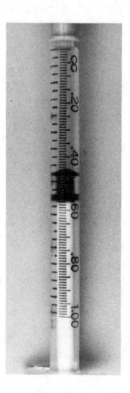 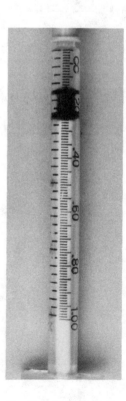

1. _____   2. _____   3. _____

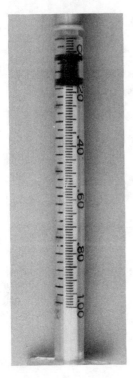

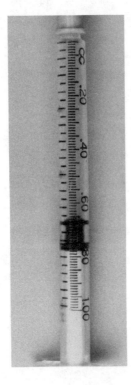

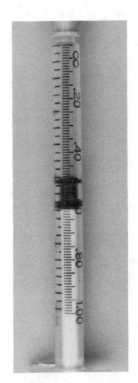

4. _____   5. _____   6. _____

ANSWERS: **1.** 0.24 cc   **2.** 0.46 cc   **3.** 0.15 cc   **4.** 0.06 cc   **5.** 0.67 cc   **6.** 0.50 cc

PROBLEM

Draw an arrow or shade in the barrel to identify the dosages indicated on the following TB syringes. Have your instructor check your answers.

1. 0.28 cc

2. 0.61 cc

3. 0.45 cc

4. 0.12 cc

5. 0.97 cc

6. 0.70 cc

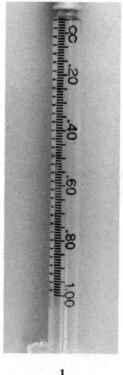

1

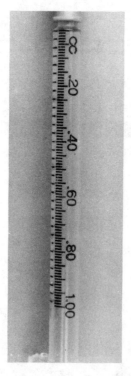

2

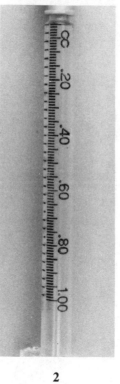

3

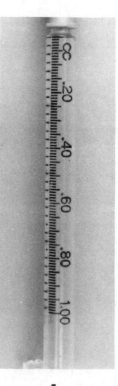

4

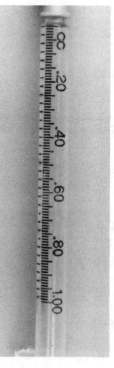

5

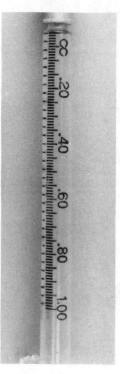

6

• TUBEX® AND CARPUJECT® CARTRIDGES •

Tubex® and Carpuject® are the trade names of the two most widely used injection cartridges. These cartridges come pre-filled with sterile medication and are clearly labeled to identify both drug and dosage. The cartridges are designed to slip into plastic injectors, which provide the plunger for the actual injection. Refer to the Tubex® cartridge in figure 26, and the Carpuject® cartridge in figure 27.

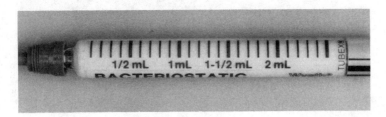

Figure 26

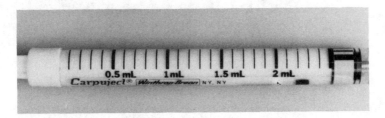

Figure 27

As you can see both cartridges have a volume of 2.5 mL. They are calibrated in tenths, and each 0.5 (½) mL has a heavier calibration, which is also numbered. The cartridges are routinely overfilled with 0.1 mL to 0.2 mL of medication to allow for manipulation of the syringe to expel air from the needle prior to injection. The cartridges are designed with sufficient capacity to allow for addition of a second drug when combined dosages are ordered. An example would be a pain medication of meperidine 75 mg in a cartridge to which Vistaril 50 mg is added.

PROBLEM

Identify the dosages measured on the following cartridges.

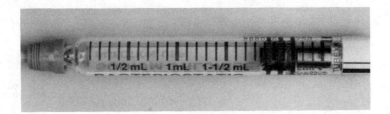

1. _____

2. _____

3. _____

4. _____

5. _____

6. _____

PROBLEM

Shade in the cartridges to indicate the following dosages. Have your instructor double check your answers.

1. 2.5 mL

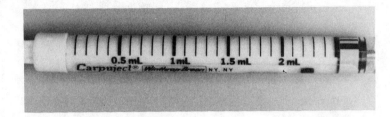

2. 1.4 mL

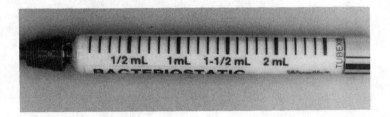

3. The cartridge contains 1 mL of medication and you are adding 0.8 mL of a second drug.

   Total Volume _____

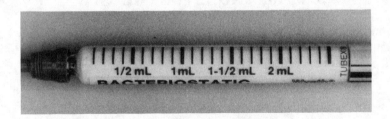

4. The cartridge contains 0.8 mL, and you must add an additional 0.8 mL.

   Total Volume _____

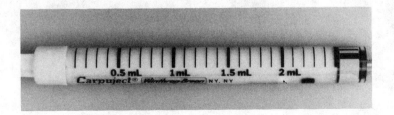

5. The cartridge contain 1.5 mL, and you are to add another 1 mL.

   Total Volume _____

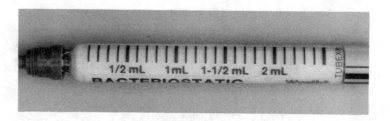

6. The cartridge contains 1 mL, and you must add an additional 1.2 mL.

   Total Volume _____

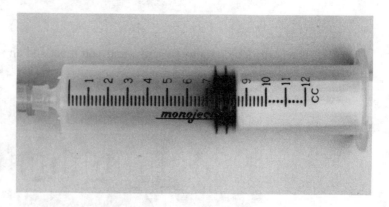

ANSWERS   3. 1.8 mL   **4.** 1.6 mL   **5.** 2.5 mL   **6.** 2.2 mL

• 5, 6, 10, AND 12 cc SYRINGES •

When volumes larger than 3 cc are required a 5, 6, 10 or 12 cc syringe may be used. Refer to figure 28 and examine the calibrations between each numbered cc to determine how these syringes are calibrated.

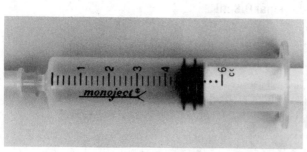
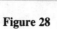

Figure 28

As you have discovered the calibrations divide each cc of these syringes into five, so that each shorter calibration actually measures two tenths, 0.2 cc. The 6 cc syringe on the left measures 4.6 cc, and the 12 cc syringe on the right measures 7.4 cc. These syringes are most often used to measure whole rather than fractional cc's, but in your practice readings we will include a full range of measurements.

PROBLEM

What dosages are measured on the following syringes?

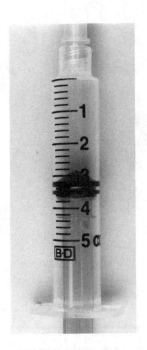

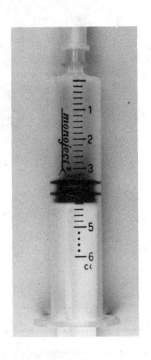

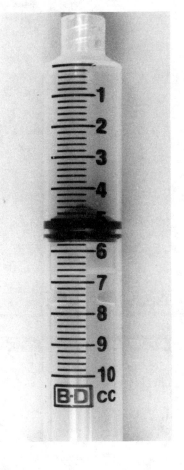

1. _____

2. _____

3. _____

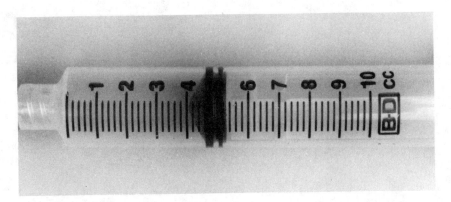

4. _____

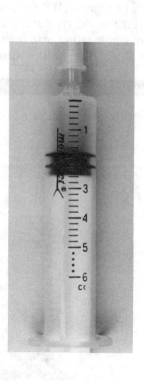

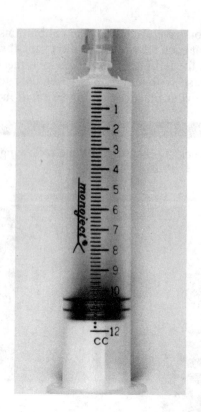

5. _____   6. _____

PROBLEM

Measure the dosages indicated on the following syringes. Have an instructor double check your accuracy.

1. 1.4 cc

2. 3.2 cc

3. 6.8 cc

4. 9.4 cc

5. 3 cc

6. 5.6 cc

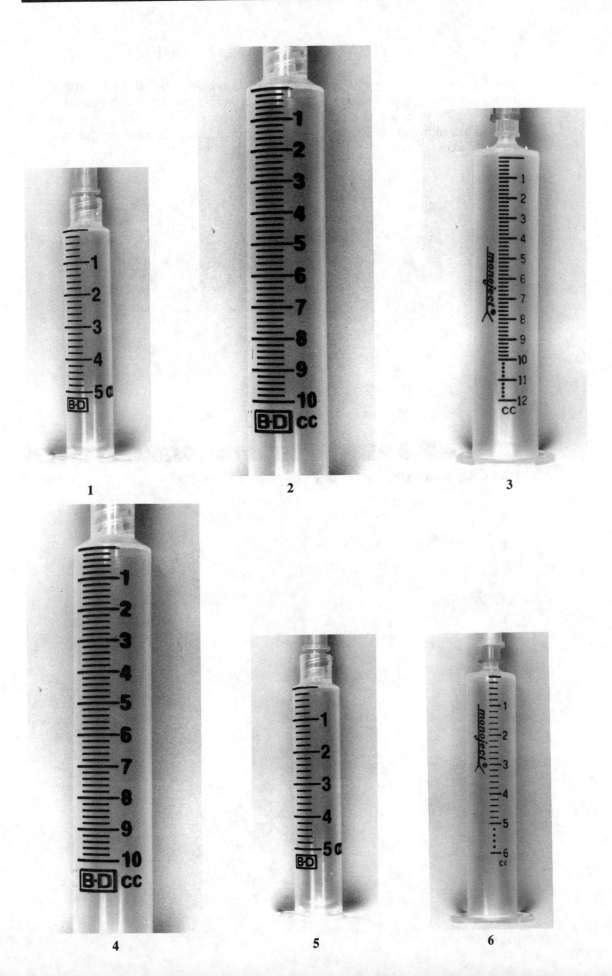

1

2

3

4

5

6

• SYRINGES 20 cc AND LARGER •

Examine the 20 cc syringe in figure 29 and determine how it is calibrated. You will notice that this syringe is calibrated in 1 cc increments, with larger calibrations identifying the 0, 5, 10, 15 and 20 cc volumes. Syringes with a 50 cc capacity are also calibrated in full cc measures. Use these syringes only for measurement of large volumes.

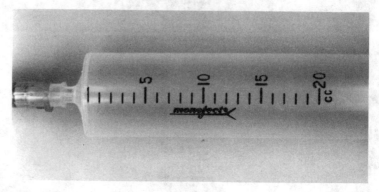

Figure 29

PROBLEM

What dosages are measured on the following 20 cc syringes?

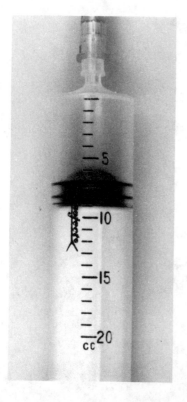

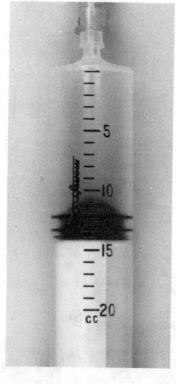

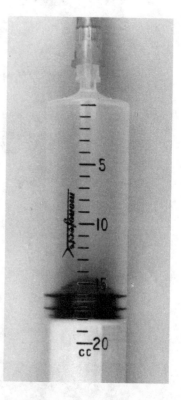

1. _____   2. _____   3. _____

PROBLEM

Shade in or draw arrows on the following syringe barrels to identify the following volumes. Have your answers double checked.

1. 11 cc

2. 18 cc

3. 9 cc

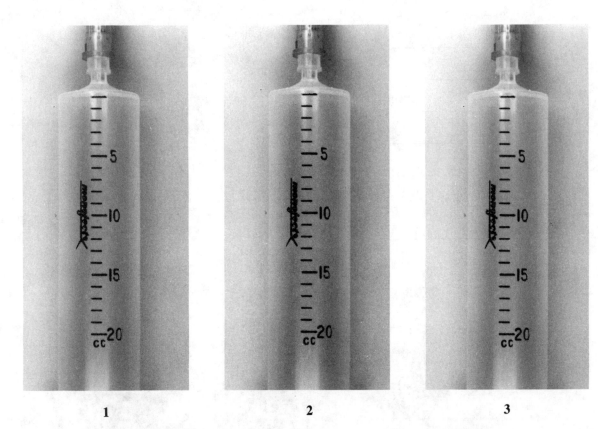

1   2   3

    This concludes your introduction to syringe calibrations. The important points to remember from this chapter are:

- 3 cc syringes are calibrated in tenths
- TB syringes are calibrated in hundredths
- 5, 6, 10 and 12 cc syringes are calibrated in fifths
- syringes larger than 12 cc are calibrated in full cc measures
- the first long calibration on all syringes indicates zero
- pre-filled cartridges such as the Tubex® and Carpuject® are overfilled with 0.1–0.2 mL of medication to allow for air expulsion from the needle
- pre-filled cartridges are sufficiently large to allow for addition of a second compatible drug
- all syringe calibrations must be read from the top, or front ring of the plunger's suction cup

Hypodermic Syringe Measurement

DIRECTIONS Identify the dosages measured on the following syringes and cartridges.

1. _____

2. _____

3. _____

4. _____

5. _____

6. _____

7. _____

8. _____

9. _____

10. _____

11. _____

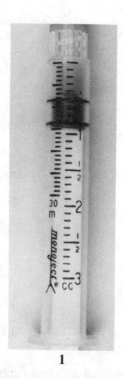

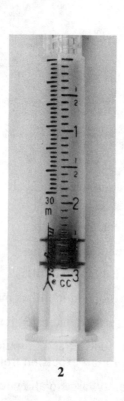

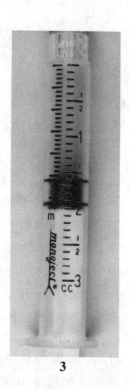

1   2   3

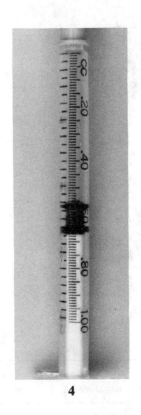

4

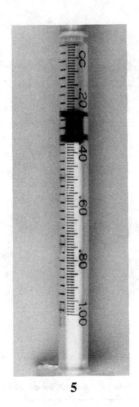

5

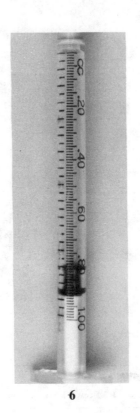

6

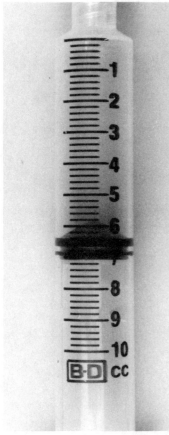

7

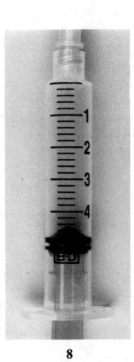

8

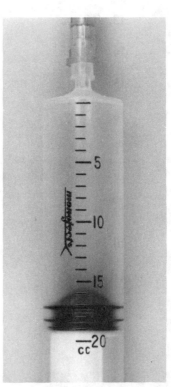

9

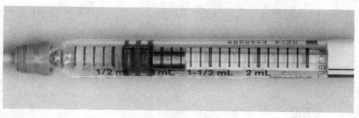

10

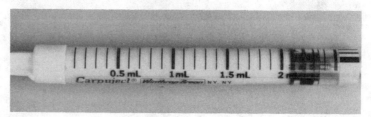

11

DIRECTIONS Draw arrows or shade the barrels on the following syringes/cartridges to measure the indicated dosages. Have your answers double checked.

12. 0.52 cc

13. 0.31 cc

14. 0.94 cc

15. 13 cc

16. 1.2 cc

17. 7.6 cc

18. 1.1 mL

19. 0.7 mL

20. 1.7 cc

21. 2.2 cc

22. 0.9 cc

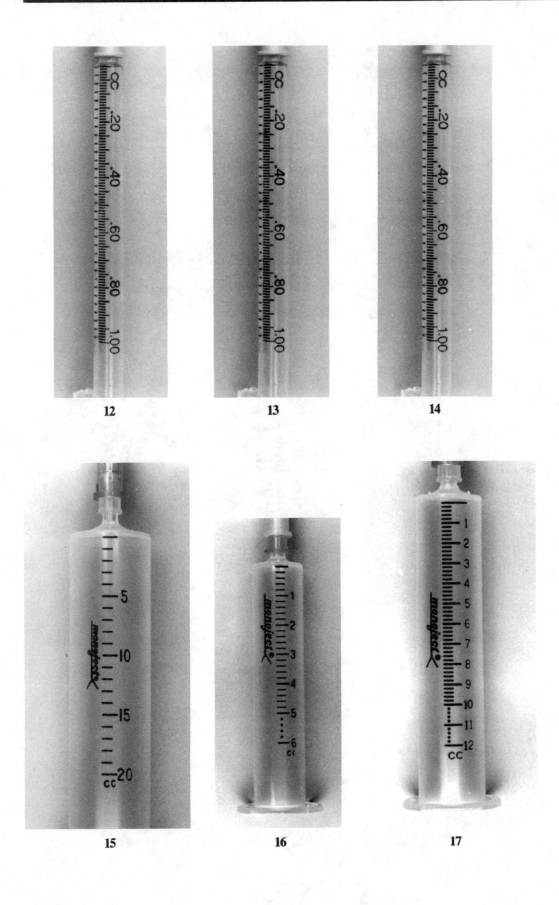

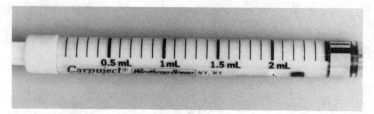

18

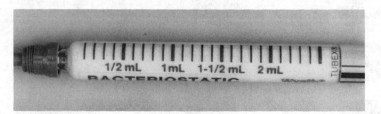

19

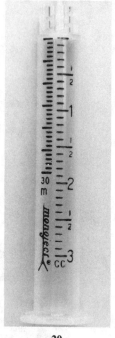

20

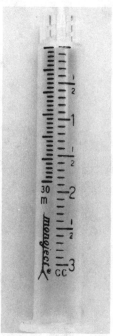

21

22

11
Reading Parenteral Medication Labels

OBJECTIVES
The student will demonstrate ability to
1. read parenteral solution labels and identify dosage strengths
2. identify milliequivalents and International Units as drug dosage measurements
3. measure parenteral dosages in metric, apothecary, milliequivalent, unit, percentage, and ratio strengths using a 3 cc syringe

INTRODUCTION
Parenteral medications are administered by injection, the intravenous (IV), intramuscular (IM), and subcutaneous (s.c.) being the most frequently used routes. The labels of oral and parenteral solutions are very similar, but the volume of the average parenteral dosage is much smaller. Intramuscular and subcutaneous solutions in particular are manufactured so that the **average adult dosage will be contained in a volume of between 1 and 3 mL**. Volumes larger than 3 mL are difficult for a single injection site to absorb, while dosages contained in a volume of less than 1 mL may require the use of a tuberculin syringe to prepare accurately. The 1–3 mL volume can be used as a guideline for accuracy of calculations in IM and s.c. dosages. Excessively larger or smaller volumes would need to be questioned, and calculations rechecked.

Intravenous medication administration is usually a two step procedure: the dosage is prepared first, then further diluted prior to administration. In this chapter we will be concerned only with the first step of IV drug preparation, which is accurate measurement of the prescribed dosage.

Parenteral drugs are packaged in a variety of single use ampules, single and multiple use rubber stoppered vials and increasingly, in pre-measured syringes and cartridges. See figure 30.

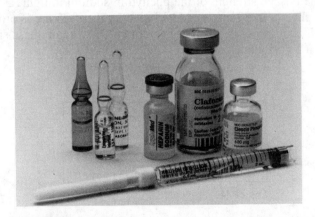

Figure 30

• READING SOLUTION LABELS •

We will begin by looking at parenteral solution labels on which the dosages are expressed in metric, apothecary, percentage and ratio strengths, since these measures are now familiar to you.

EXAMPLE 1   Refer to the Vistaril® label in figure 31. The immediate difference you will notice between this and oral solution labels is the size. Ampules and vials are small and their labels are small, which requires that they be read with particular care. The information however, is similar to oral labels. Vistaril® is the trade name of the drug, hydroxyzine HCl is the generic name. The dosage strength is 100 mg per 2 cc. Calculating dosages is not usually complicated. For example if a dosage of Vistaril® 100 mg is ordered you would give 2 cc, if 50 mg are ordered give 1 cc, for 25 mg give 0.5 cc.

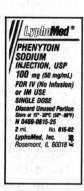

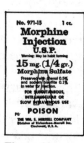

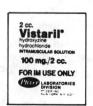

Figure 31   Figure 32   Figure 33

EXAMPLE 2   The morphine sulfate solution in figure 32 has a dosage strength of 15 mg per cc (gr ¼ per cc). Notice that the label lists the weight under the drug name, but that you must locate the volume which contains this weight elsewhere (upper right corner). Ampules are frequently labeled in this manner.

To administer 15 mg of morphine you would give 1 cc. To obtain a dosage of 8 mg give 0.5 cc. Give 1 cc for gr ¼, and 0.5 cc for gr ⅛.

EXAMPLE 3   The dosage strength of the phenytoin sodium in figure 33 is 50 mg/mL. If phenytoin 50 mg is ordered give 1 mL, if 25 mg is ordered give 0.5 mL, if 100 mg is ordered give 2 mL. Once again these simple dosages can be calculated mentally.

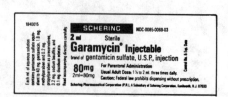

Figure 34

PROBLEM

Refer to the gentamicin label in figure 34 and answer the following questions.

1. What is the total volume of this vial? _____

2. What is the dosage strength? _____

3. If gentamicin 80 mg were ordered how many mL would this be? _____

4. If gentamicin 60 mg were ordered how many mL would this be? _____

5. How many mL would you need to prepare a 20 mg dosage? _____

ANSWERS   **1.** 2 mL   **2.** 2 mL = 80 mg   **3.** 2 mL   **4.** 1.5 mL   **5.** 0.5 mL

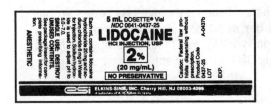

Figure 35

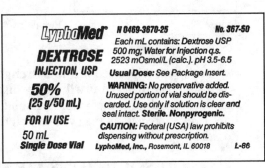

Figure 36

Drugs labeled as **percentage solutions** also often express the drug strength in metric measures. Refer to the lidocaine label in figure 35. Notice that this is a 2% solution, and the vial which contains it has a total volume of 5 mL. Also notice that the dosage strength is listed in metric measures: 20 mg/mL. Lidocaine is most often ordered in mg, for example 20 mg requires 1 mL, 10 mg would require 0.5 mL, and 30 mg would require 1.5 mL. However, lidocaine is also used as a local anesthetic and a doctor may request for example, that you prepare 3 mL of 2% lidocaine, which requires no calculation at all, but simply locating the correct percentage strength, and drawing up 3 mL. **Dosages prescribed or requested by their percentage strength will state the number of mL/cc to prepare.**

PROBLEM

Refer to the dextrose label in figure 36 and answer the following questions.

1. What is the percentage strength of this dextrose solution? _____

2. How many mL does the vial contain? _____

3. If you are asked to prepare 20 mL of a 50% dextrose solution how much will you

draw up in the syringe? _____

4. The dosage also appears on this label in metric measures. What is the metric dosage strength of this solution? _____

5. If you are asked to prepare 25 g of dextrose from this vial what volume will you draw up? _____

ANSWERS   **1.** 50%   **2.** 50 mL   **3.** 20 mL   **4.** 25 g/50 mL   **5.** 50 mL

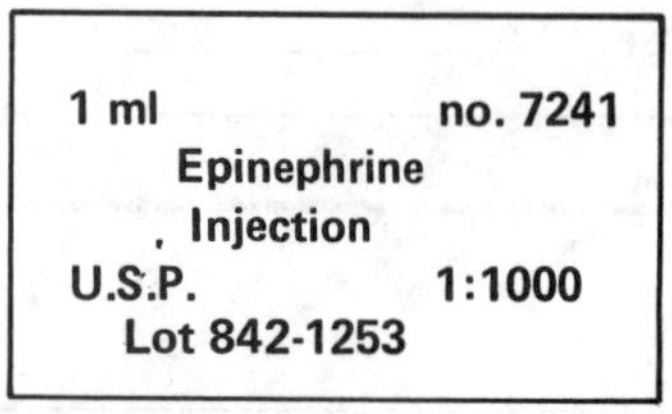

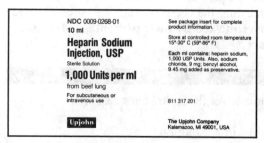

Figure 37

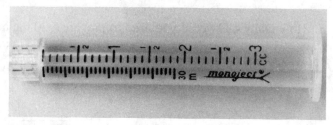

Figure 38

Solutions expressed in **ratio strengths** are becoming much less common, but **when they are ordered it will be by number of cc/mL**. Refer to figure 37. Notice that the strength of this epinephrine solution is 1:1000, and that the ampule contains only 1 mL. Indicate on the syringe in figure 38 how you would prepare a 0.8 mL dosage.

• SOLUTIONS MEASURED IN UNITS (u) •

Many drugs are measured in **International Units**. Insulin, penicillin and heparin are examples of drugs commonly measured in units. A unit measures a drug in terms of its action, not its physical weight. Units may be abbreviated **u**, and are expressed using Arabic numerals with the abbreviation following, for example 2,000 u, or 1,000,000 u.

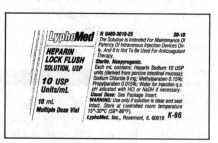

Figure 39

Figure 40

PROBLEM

1. What is the dosage strength of the heparin solution in figure 39? _____

2. If you are to prepare a dosage of 500 u what volume will you need?

   _____

_____

ANSWERS   **1.** 1,000 u/mL   **2.** 0.5 mL

PROBLEM

1. What is the strength of the heparin solution in figure 40? _____

2. If 10 u are ordered to flush a heplock, what volume will you prepare?

   _____

_____

ANSWERS   **1.** 10 u/mL   **2.** 1 mL

PROBLEM

Refer to the heparin label in figure 41 and answer the following questions.

1. What is the total volume of this vial? _____

2. What is the dosage strength? _____

3. If a volume of 1.5 mL is prepared how many units will this be? _____

4. How many mL will you need to give a dosage of 55,000 u? _____

5. If 0.25 mL of this medication is prepared what dosage will this be?

   _____

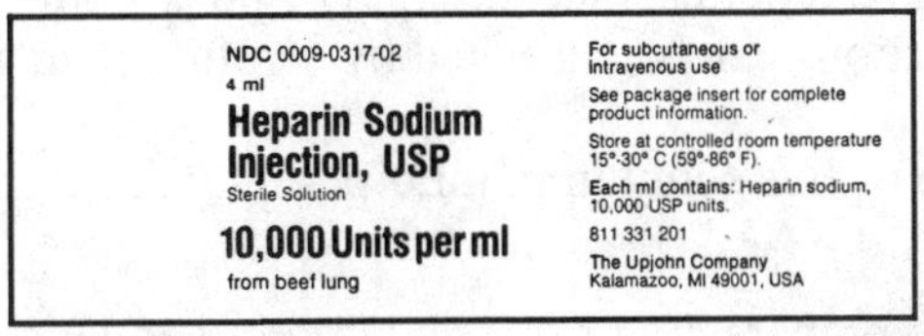

NDC 0009-0317-02
4 ml

Heparin Sodium Injection, USP
Sterile Solution

10,000 Units per ml
from beef lung

For subcutaneous or intravenous use

See package insert for complete product information.

Store at controlled room temperature 15°-30° C (59°-86° F).

Each ml contains: Heparin sodium, 10,000 USP units.

811 331 201
The Upjohn Company
Kalamazoo, MI 49001, USA

Figure 41

_____

ANSWERS   **1.** 4 mL   **2.** 10,000 u/mL   **3.** 15,000 u   **4.** 5.5 mL   **5.** 2500 u

• SOLUTIONS MEASURED AS
MILLIEQUIVALENTS (mEq) •

Milliequivalents (mEq) is an expression of the number of grams of a drug contained in 1 mL of a normal solution. This is a definition which will be quite understandable to a pharmacist, but you need not memorize it. Refer to the calcium gluconate label in figure 42 and notice that this solution has a dosage strength of 0.465 mEq/mL. If a dosage of 0.465 mEq were ordered you would draw up 1 mL in the syringe.

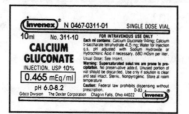

Figure 42

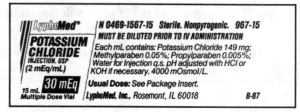

Figure 43

PROBLEM

Refer to the potassium chloride label in figure 43 and answer the following questions.

1. What is the total volume and total dosage strength of this vial? _____

2. What is the dosage in mEq per mL? _____

3. If you are asked to prepare 30 mEq for addition to an IV what volume would you
   draw up? _____

ANSWERS   1. 15 mL/30 mEq   2. 2 mEq/mL   3. 15 mL

PROBLEM

Refer to the potassium chloride label in figure 44, and answer the following dosage questions. Notice that this label lists the strength of potassium chloride in mg as well as mEq. All of the questions can be answered by careful reading of the label.

1. What is the strength of this solution in mEq per mL? _____

2. If you were asked to prepare 40 mEq for addition to an IV solution what volume
   would you draw up in the syringe? _____

3. What is the strength of this solution expressed in mg per mL? _____

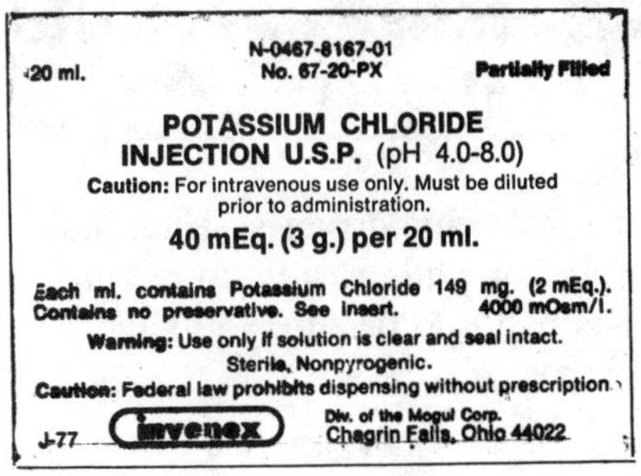

Figure 44

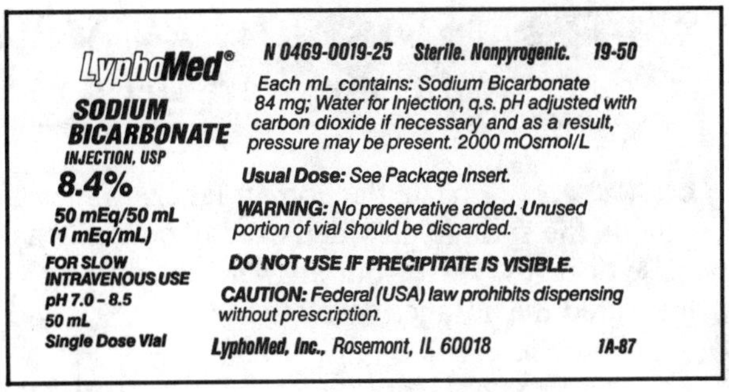

Figure 45

ANSWERS   **1.** 2 mEq/mL   **2.** 20 mL   **3.** 149 mg

PROBLEM

Refer to the sodium bicarbonate label in figure 45. Notice that this solution lists the drug strength in mEq, percentage, and mg. Read the label very carefully and locate the answers to the following questions.

1. What is the dosage strength expressed in mEq/mL? _____

2. What is the total volume of the vial, and how many mEq does this volume contain? _____

3. What is the strength per mL expressed as mg? _____

4. If you were asked to prepare 10 mL of an 8.4% sodium bicarbonate solution, what volume would you draw up in a syringe? _____

ANSWERS   **1.** 1 mEq/mL   **2.** 50 mL/50 mEq   **3.** 84 mg/mL   **4.** 10 mL

This concludes the introduction to parenteral solution labels. The important points to remember from this chapter are:

- the most commonly used parenteral administration routes are IV, IM, and s.c.

- the labels of most parenteral solutions are quite small and must be read with particular care

- the average IM and s.c. dosage will be contained in a volume of between 1 and 3 mL. This volume can be used as a guideline to accuracy of calculations

- IV medication preparation is usually a two step procedure: measurement of the dosage, then dilution according to manufacturers recommendations or doctors order

- parenteral drugs may be measured in metric, apothecary, ratio, percentage, unit or mEq dosages

- if dosages are ordered by percentage or ratio strength they are usually specified in cc/mL to be administered

- most IM and s.c. dosages are prepared using a 3 cc or 1 cc tuberculin syringe

Reading Parenteral Medication Labels

DIRECTIONS Locate the correct labels to measure the following dosages. Then indicate on the syringe provided exactly how much solution you will draw up to obtain these dosages. Have your answers checked by your instructor to be sure you have measured the dosages correctly.

Dosage Ordered	**mL/cc Needed**

1. Depo-Provera® 0.2 g   _____

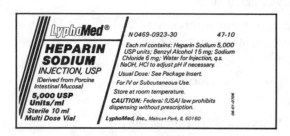

NDC 0009-0248-02
5 ml Vial
Depo-Provera®
Sterile Aqueous Suspension
sterile medroxyprogesterone
acetate suspension, USP
100 mg per ml

For intramuscular use only
See package insert for complete
product information.
Shake vigorously immediately
before each use.
Store at controlled room temperature
15°-30° C (59°-86° F)
811 851 201
The Upjohn Company
Kalamazoo, Michigan 49001, USA

2. furosemide 10 mg   _____

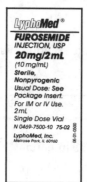

LyphoMed®
FUROSEMIDE
INJECTION, USP
20 mg/2 mL
(10 mg/mL)
Sterile,
Nonpyrogenic
Usual Dose: See
Package Insert.
For IM or IV Use.
2 mL
Single Dose Vial
N 0469-7500-10 75-02
LyphoMed, Inc.
Melrose Park, IL 60160

3. heparin 2,500 u   _____

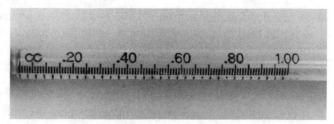

LyphoMed®
**HEPARIN
SODIUM**
INJECTION, USP
(Derived from Porcine
Intestinal Mucosa)
**5,000 USP
Units/ml**
Sterile 10 ml
Multi Dose Vial

N 0469-0923-30   47-10
Each ml contains: Heparin Sodium 5,000
USP units; Benzyl Alcohol 15 mg; Sodium
Chloride 6 mg; Water for Injection, q.s.
NaOH, HCl to adjust pH if necessary.
Usual Dose: See Package Insert.
For IV or Subcutaneous Use.
Store at room temperature.
CAUTION: Federal (USA) law prohibits
dispensing without prescription.
LyphoMed, Inc., Melrose Park, IL 60160

4. Cleocin® 0.9 g _____

NDC 0009-0902-11   6 ml Vial

LOT
EXP

Cleocin Phosphate®
Sterile Solution
clindamycin phosphate
injection, USP

900 mg

Equivalent to 900 mg clindamycin

Single Dose Container

See package insert for complete
product information.

Store at controlled room
temperature 15°-30° C
(59°-86° F)

812 823 103

The Upjohn Company
Kalamazoo, MI 49001, USA

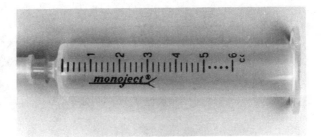

5. atropine 0.2 mg _____

20 mL Multiple Dose Vial
NDC 0641-2210-41
6505-00-754-2547

ATROPINE
SULFATE INJECTION, USP

400 mcg/mL
(0.4 mg/mL)
FOR SC, IM OR IV USE

Each mL contains atropine sulfate
400 mcg (0.4 mg), sodium chloride
9 mg and benzyl alcohol 0.015 mL in
Water for Injection. pH 3.0-6.5;
sulfuric acid added, if needed, for
pH adjustment.

POISON

Usual Dose: See package insert.
Store at controlled room tem-
perature 15°-30° C (59°-86° F).
Caution: Federal law prohibits
dispensing without prescription.
Product Code
2210-41
LOT   EXP.

A-2210t

Table of Equivalents			
mcg	mg	mL	
100	0.1	0.25	
120	0.12	0.3	
160	0.16	0.4	
200	0.2	0.5	
240	0.24	0.6	
320	0.32	0.8	
400	0.4	1.0	
600	0.6	1.5	
800	0.8	2.0	

esi **ELKINS-SINN, INC. Cherry Hill, NJ 08003-4099**
A subsidiary of A. H. Robins Company

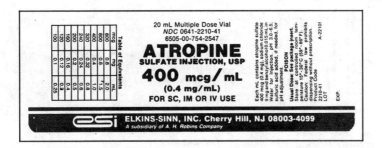

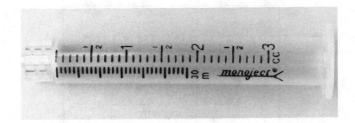

6. seconal gr ¾ _____

20 cc.   **AMPOULE No. 616**

SECONAL'
SODIUM
SODIUM SECOBARBITAL INJECTION
50 mg. (3/4 gr.) per cc.
WARNING—May be habit forming.
For Use as a Basal Hypnotic

REFRIGERATE *Lilly*
XG 7722   AMX
ELI LILLY & CO., INDIANAPOLIS, U.S.A.

CAUTION: Federal (U.S.A.) law prohibits dispensing without prescription.
Each cc. contains SECONAL Sodium 50 mg.
(3/4 gr.) in Sterile Water for Injection with
Polyethylene Glycol 50%. Phenol
0.25%. Sodium hydroxide and/or hydrochloric
acid may have been added during manufacture
to adjust pH.
Improper storage may cause precipitation. Return Ampoule.
Note: Suitable for both intramuscular and intravenous injection as described in literature.

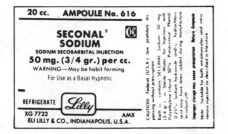

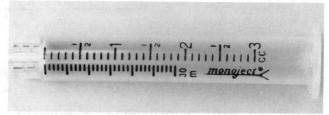

7. Robinul® 100 mcg _____

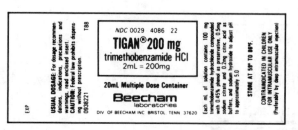

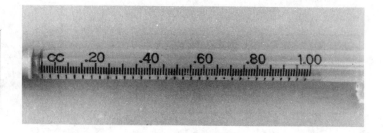

8. Tigan® 200 mg _____

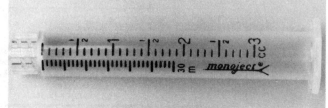

9. aminophylline 0.25 g _____

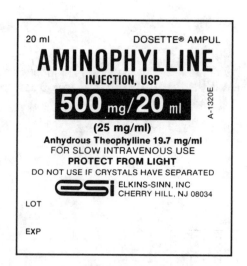

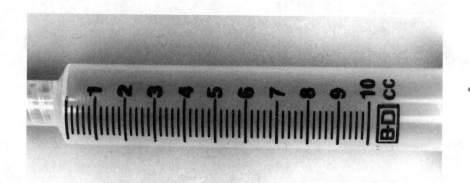

10. cyanocobalamin 1000 mcg   _____

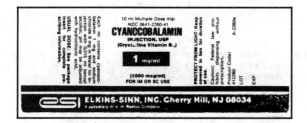
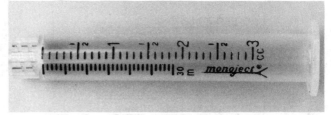

11. fentanyl 0.125 mg   _____

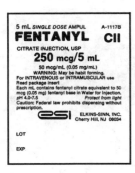
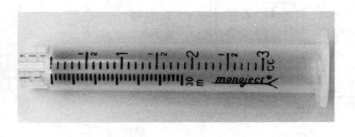

12. amikacin 100 mg   _____

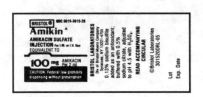
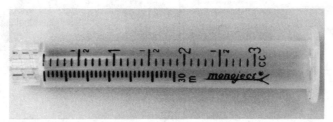

13. Zantac 75 mg   _____

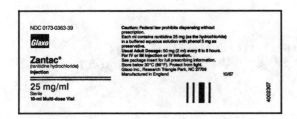
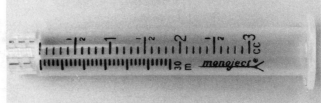

14.   calcium gluconate 0.93 mEq   _____

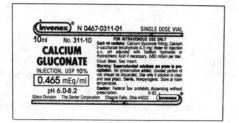
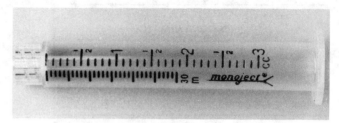

15.   diazepam 7.5 mg   _____

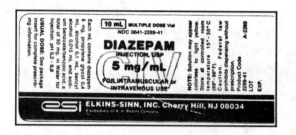
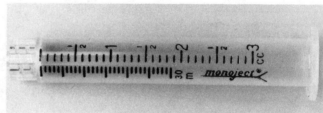

16.   heparin 1000 u   _____

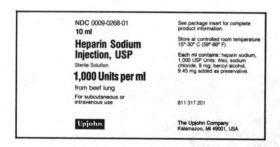
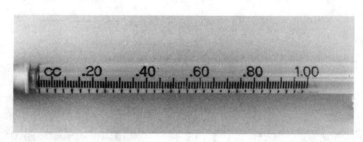

17.   perphenazine 2.5 mg   _____

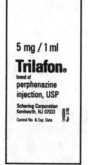
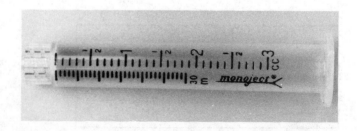

18. phenytoin Na 0.15 g _____

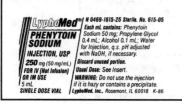
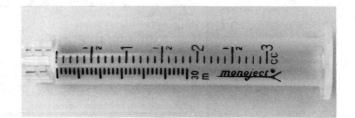

19. medroxyprogesterone 1 g _____

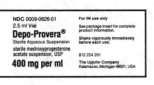
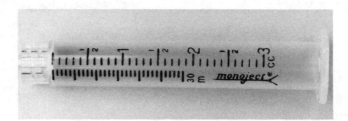

20. gentamicin 60 mg _____

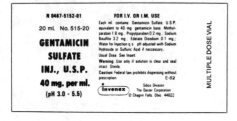
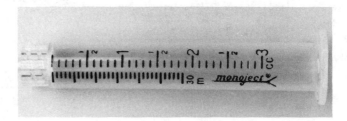

21. lidocaine 1% 5 mL _____

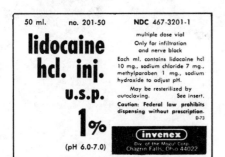
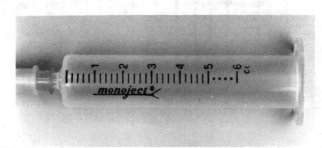

22. sodium acetate 20 mEq   _____

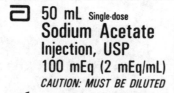

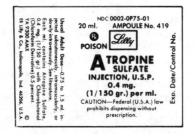

23. atropine gr ¹⁄₁₅₀   _____

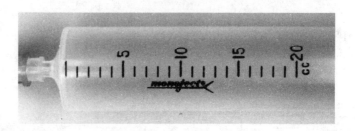

24. meperidine 50 mg   _____

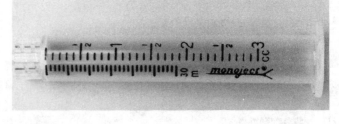

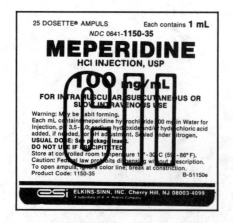

25. Aristospan® 20 mg _____

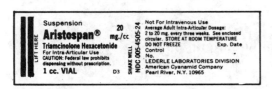

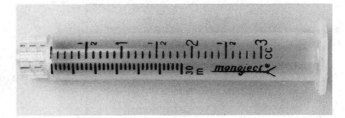

Suspension
Aristospan® 20 mg./cc
Triamcinolone Hexacetonide
For Intra-Articular Use
CAUTION: Federal law prohibits
dispensing without prescription.
1 cc. VIAL   D3

Not For Intravenous Use:
Average Adult Intra-Articular Dosage:
2 to 20 mg. every three weeks. See enclosed
circular. STORE AT ROOM TEMPERATURE
DO NOT FREEZE   Exp. Date
Control
No.
LEDERLE LABORATORIES DIVISION
American Cyanamid Company
Pearl River, N.Y. 10965

NDC 005-4505-24   SHAKE WELL   LIFT HERE

26. clindamycin 0.3 g _____

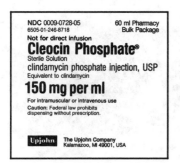

NDC 0009-0728-05   60 ml Pharmacy
6505-01-246-8718   Bulk Package
Not for direct infusion
Cleocin Phosphate®
Sterile Solution
clindamycin phosphate injection, USP
Equivalent to clindamycin
150 mg per ml
For intramuscular or intravenous use
Caution: Federal law prohibits
dispensing without prescription.

Upjohn   The Upjohn Company
Kalamazoo, MI 49001, USA

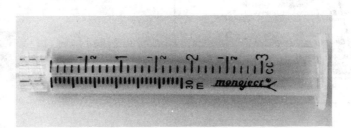

27. morphine sulfate 15 mg _____

20 mL Multiple Dose Vial
NDC 0641-2345-41
MORPHINE
SULFATE INJECTION, USP
15 mg/mL
FOR SUBCUTANEOUS,
INTRAMUSCULAR OR SLOW
INTRAVENOUS USE
NOT FOR EPIDURAL
OR INTRATHECAL USE

Each mL contains morphine sulfate
15 mg, (WARNING: May be habit forming)
sodium phosphate, monobasic
sodium phosphate, anhydrous 2.8
mg, sodium formaldehyde sulfoxylate 3 mg and phenol 2.5 mg
Water for Injection, pH 2.5-6.0;
sulfuric acid added, if needed, for
pH adjustment. Sealed under nitrogen.
USUAL DOSE: See package insert.

DO NOT USE IF PRECIPITATED
PROTECT FROM LIGHT
NOTE: Slight discoloration will not
alter efficacy. Discard if markedly
discolored.
Store at controlled room temper-
ature 15°-30°C (59°-86°F)
Caution: Federal law prohibits
dispensing without prescription.
Product Code: 2345-41   A-2345
LOT
EXP

esi   **ELKINS-SINN, INC. Cherry Hill, NJ 08034**
A subsidiary of A. H. Robins Company

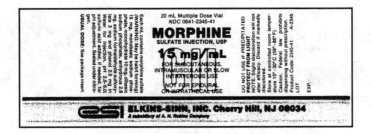

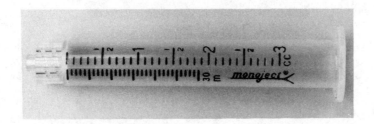

28. lincomycin HCl 0.6 g _____

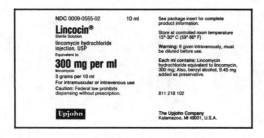

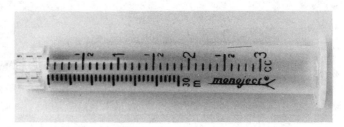

29. nitroglycerin 10 mg _____

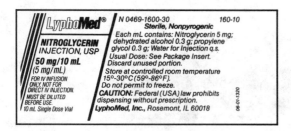

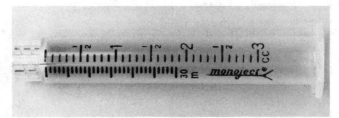

30. hydroxyzine HCl 0.1 g _____

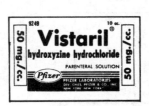

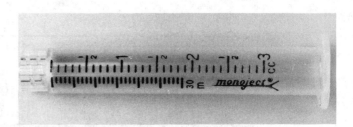

31. meperidine 50 mg _____

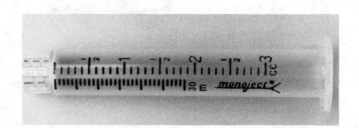

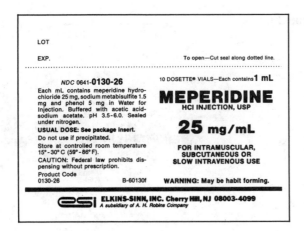

Label: NDC 0641-0130-26 MEPERIDINE HCl INJECTION, USP 25 mg/mL. 10 DOSETTE® VIALS—Each contains 1 mL. Each mL contains meperidine hydrochloride 25 mg, sodium metabisulfite 1.5 mg and phenol 5 mg in Water for Injection. Buffered with acetic acid-sodium acetate. pH 3.5-6.0. Sealed under nitrogen. USUAL DOSE: See package insert. Do not use if precipitated. Store at controlled room temperature 15°-30°C (59°-86°F). CAUTION: Federal law prohibits dispensing without prescription. Product Code 0130-26   B-60130f. FOR INTRAMUSCULAR, SUBCUTANEOUS OR SLOW INTRAVENOUS USE. WARNING: May be habit forming. ELKINS-SINN, INC. Cherry Hill, NJ 08003-4099 A subsidiary of A. H. Robins Company.

32. methadone HCl 15 mg   _____

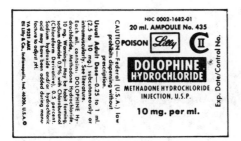

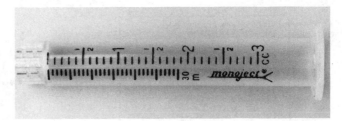

33. Celestone® 12 mg   _____

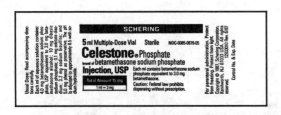

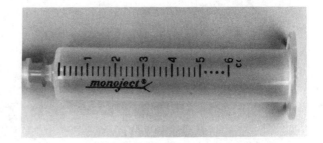

34. naloxone 0.8 mg   _____

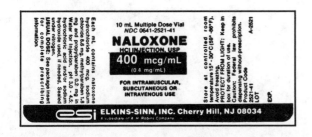

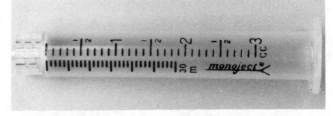

35. dexamethasone 2 mg _____

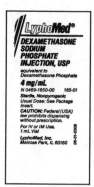

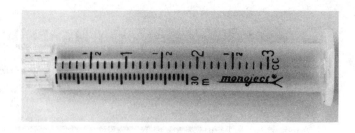

36. Vesprin® 15 mg _____

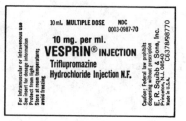

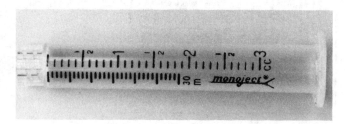

37. Pronestyl® 0.5 g _____

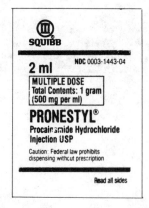

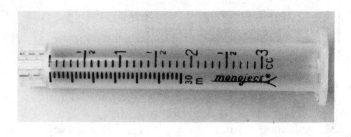

38. hydroxyzine HCl 50 mg _____

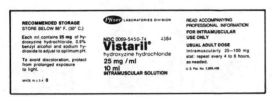

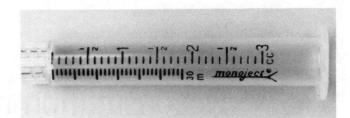

39. morphine 15 mg _____

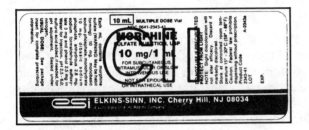

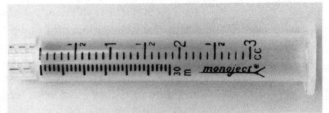

40. Betalin® 0.2 mg _____

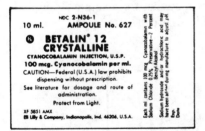

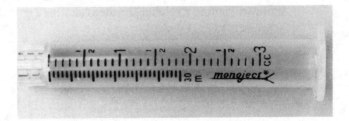

ANSWERS

1. 2 mL **2.** 1 mL **3.** 0.5 mL **4.** 6 mL **5.** 0.5 mL **6.** 1 cc **7.** 0.5 mL **8.** 2 mL **9.** 10 mL **10.** 1 mL **11.** 2.5 mL **12.** 2 ml
13. 3 mL **14.** 2 mL **15.** 1.5 mL **16.** 1 mL **17.** 0.5 mL **18.** 3 mL **19.** 2.5 mL **20.** 1.5 mL **21.** 5 mL **22.** 10 mL **23.** 1 mL
24. 0.5 mL **25.** 1 cc **26.** 2 mL **27.** 1 mL **28.** 2 mL **29.** 2 mL **30.** 2 cc **31.** 2 mL **32.** 1.5 mL **33.** 4 mL **34.** 2 mL
35. 0.5 mL **36.** 1.5 mL **37.** 1 mL **38.** 2 mL **39.** 1.5 mL **40.** 2 mL

12
Reconstitution of Powdered Drugs

OBJECTIVES
The student will
1. prepare solutions from powdered drugs using directions printed on vial labels
2. prepare solutions from powdered drugs using drug literature or inserts
3. determine expiration dates and times for reconstituted drugs
4. calculate simple dosages from reconstituted drugs

INTRODUCTION
Many drugs are shipped in powdered form because they retain their potency only a short time in solution. Reconstitution of these drugs is often the responsibility of hospital pharmacies, but this does not eliminate the need for nurses to know how to read and follow reconstitution directions, and how to label drugs with an expiration date and time once they have been reconstituted. The drug label or instructional package insert will give specific directions for reconstitution of the drug. Reading these requires care and this chapter will take you step by step through the entire process.

• RECONSTITUTION OF A SINGLE STRENGTH SOLUTION •

Let's start with the simplest type of reconstitution instructions, for a single strength solution. Examine the label for the oxacillin 2 g vial in figure 46.

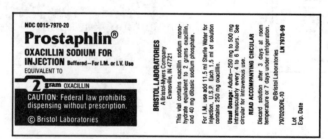

Figure 46

The first step in reconstitution is to locate the directions. They are on this label at the right side, printed sideways. Notice that the instructions read "for IM use add 11.5 mL sterile water." This would be done using a sterile syringe and aseptic technique. The vial is then agitated until all the powder has dissolved.

Next notice the information which relates to the length of time the reconstituted solution may be stored. You are instructed to "discard solution after 3 days at room temperature, or 7 days under refrigeration." **The person mixing a solution is responsible for printing her or his initials on the vial, as well as the time and date of expiration**, unless all the drug is used when initially mixed. If the solution above was mixed at 2 p.m. on January 3rd, what expiration information would you print on the vial if it is stored in the refrigerator? "Expires Jan 10th 2 p.m.," which is 7 days from the time mixed. If it is stored at room temperature it must be labeled "Expires Jan 6th 2 p.m.," which is 3 days.

Once the solution is prepared and labeled with your initials and the expiration date, you can concentrate on the dosage strength. Notice that the label indicates that "Each 1.5 mL of solution contains 250 mg oxacillin." There is a total dosage of 2 g in this vial, or eight dosages of 250 mg at 1.5 mL each, for a total volume of 12 mL. You added only 11.5 mL to the vial to reconstitute the drug, and the reason for the increased volume is that the powder itself occupies space. **The total volume of the prepared solution will always exceed the volume of the diluent you add**, because it consists of the diluent plus the powder volume. Refer to the dosage strength again, which is 250 mg per 1.5 mL. If a 250 mg dosage is ordered you would prepare 1.5 mL; for a 0.5 g dosage prepare 3 mL.

PROBLEM

Another medication prepared in powdered form is ticarcillin disodium. Refer to the label in figure 47 and answer the following questions about this medication.

1. How much diluent is added to the vial to prepare the drug for IM use?

    _____

2. What kind of solution is used as the diluent? _____

3. What is the dosage strength of the prepared solution? _____

4. If the order is for 1 g, what volume must you give? _____

5. If the order is for 500 mg, what volume must you give? _____

6. How long will this reconstituted solution retain its potency? _____

7. If you reconstitute the drug at 8 a.m. on October 23rd, what expiration information will you print on the label if the drug is to be refrigerated? _____

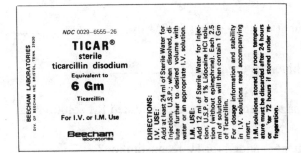

Figure 47

ANSWERS   1. 12 mL   **2.** sterile water, or Lidocaine 1% HCl   **3.** 1 Gm in 2.5 mL   **4.** 2.5 mL   **5.** 1.3 mL   **6.** 24 hrs at room temperature, or 72 hrs refrigerated   **7.** expires 8 a.m. Oct 26th

PROBLEM

Read the cefazolin 500 mg (Kefzol®) label in figure 48 and answer the following questions.

1. How much diluent is added to the vial for reconstitution? _____

2. What type of diluent is used? _____

3. What is the dosage strength of the prepared solution? _____

4. If the order is for 225 mg what volume must you give? _____

5. How long will the drug retain its potency at room temperature? _____

6. If the drug is reconstituted at 8 a.m. on Jan 3rd and stored at room temperature, what expiration date will you print on the label? _____

ANSWERS   **1.** 2 mL   **2.** sterile water, or 0.9% sodium chloride   **3.** 225 mg per mL   **4.** 1 mL   **5.** 24 hrs
6. 8 a.m. Jan 4th.

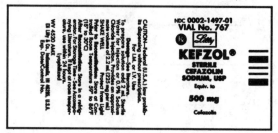

Figure 48

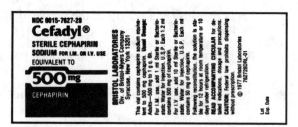

Figure 49

PROBLEM

Refer to the cephapirin 500 mg (Cefadyl®) label in figure 49 and answer the following questions.

1. How much diluent must be added for IM use? _____

2. What type of diluent is used? _____

3. What is the dosage strength of the reconstituted IM solution? _____

4. How much diluent is added for IV reconstitution? _____

5. What is the dosage strength of the reconstituted IV solution? _____

6. If the drug is reconstituted at 9 a.m. on May 10th and stored at room temperature, what expiration date and time will you print on the label? _____

7. If it is stored under refrigeration what expiration date and time will you use?

_____

ANSWERS **1.** 1 mL   **2.** sterile water   **3.** 500 mg/1.2 mL   **4.** 10 mL   **5.** 50 mg/mL   **6.** 9 p.m. May 10th
7. 9 a.m. May 20th

• RECONSTITUTION OF A MULTIPLE STRENGTH SOLUTION •

Some powdered drugs offer a choice of dosage strengths. When this is the case you must choose the strength most appropriate for the dosage ordered. For example, refer to the penicillin label in figure 50. The dosage strengths which can be obtained are listed on the left.

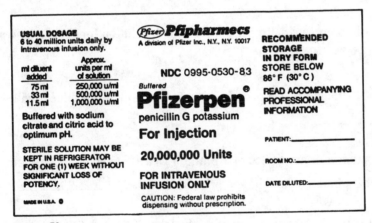

Figure 50

   If the dosage ordered is 500,000 u q.i.d., the most appropriate strength to mix would be 500,000 u per mL. Read across from this strength, and determine how much diluent must be added to obtain it. The answer is 33 mL. If the dosage ordered is 1,000,000 u q.i.d., what would be the most appropriate strength to prepare, and how much diluent would this require? The answer is 1,000,000 u/mL, and 11.5 mL.
   Notice that this label does not tell you what type of diluent to use. **When information is missing from the label look for it on the package information insert.** Don't start guessing. All the information you need is in print somewhere, just take your time and locate it.
   A multiple strength solution such as this one requires that you add one additional piece of information to the label after you reconstitute it: the dosage strength you have just mixed.

PROBLEM

If you add 75 mL of diluent to prepare a solution of penicillin from the above label, what dosage strength will you print on the label? _____

ANSWER **1.** 250,000 u/mL

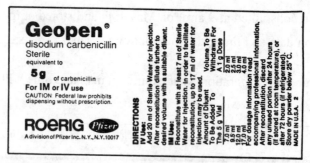

Figure 51

PROBLEM

Refer to the carbenicillin label in figure 51 and answer the following questions about reconstitution of this multiple strength medication.

1. What type of diluent is used for IV reconstitution? _____

2. What volume of diluent is used for IV reconstitution? _____

3. If you wish to prepare a 1 g per 3 mL strength solution for IM use how much diluent must you add? _____

4. If a dosage strength of 1 g per 2 mL is required how much diluent will you add? _____

5. If the solution is reconstituted at 1 p.m. on Dec 18th and stored at room temperature what expiration date will you print on the label? _____

6. What expiration date will you print on the label if the solution is refrigerated? _____

ANSWERS **1.** sterile water   **2.** 20 mL   **3.** 12 mL   **4.** 7 mL   **5.** Expires 1 p.m. Dec 19th
6. Expires 1 p.m. Dec 21st

• RECONSTITUTION FROM PACKAGE INSERT DIRECTIONS •

If the label does not contain reconstitution directions you must obtain these from the information insert which accompanies the vial. The labels for Claforan® in figures 52 and 53 fall into this category. Refer to these now, and to the portion of the package insert directions reproduced in figure 54. Notice that the insert instructions are for three vial strengths: 1 g, 2 g and 500 mg, but that only the labels for the 1 g and 2 g vials are included.

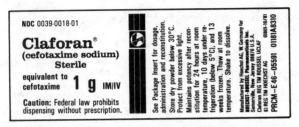

Figure 52

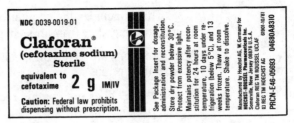

Figure 53

Preparation of Solution: Claforan for IM or IV administration should be reconstituted as follows:

Strength	Amount of Diluent To Be Added (mL)	Approximate Withdrawable Volume (mL)	Approximate Average Concentration (mg/mL)
Intramuscular			
500 mg vial	2	2.2	230
1 g vial	3	3.4	300
2 g vial	5	6.0	330
Intravenous			
500 mg vial	10	10.2	50
1 g vial	10	10.4	95
2 g vial	10	11.0	180

Shake to dissolve; inspect for particulate matter and discoloration prior to use. Solutions of Claforan range from light yellow to amber, depending on concentration, diluent used, and length and condition of storage.
For intramuscular use: Reconstitute with Sterile Water for Injection or Bacteriostatic Water for Injection as described above.

Figure 54

PROBLEM

Read the Claforan® labels and package insert provided and answer the the questions below on dosage strength and diluent quantities which pertain to them.

Vial Strength	Amount of Diluent	Dosage Strength of Prepared Solution
1. cefotaxime 1 g (prepare for IM injection)	a) _____	b) _____
2. cefotaxime 2 g (prepare for IM injection)	a) _____	b) _____
3. cefotaxime 1 g (prepare for IV administration)	a) _____	b) _____
4. cefotaxime 2 g (prepare for IV administration)	a) _____	b) _____

5. What diluent is recommended for IM reconstitution? _____

6. How long will the solution retain its potency after reconstitution?

_____

ANSWERS **1.** a) 3 mL b) 300 mg/mL **2.** a) 5 mL b) 330 mg/mL **3.** a) 10 mL b) 95 mg/mL **4.** a) 10 mL b) 180 mg/mL **5.** Sterile Water or Bacteriostatic Water **6.** 24 hours at room temperature; 10 days if refrigerated below 5°C; 13 weeks frozen

This concludes the chapter on reconstitution of powdered drugs. The important points to remember from this chapter are:

■ if directions are given on labels for both IM and IV reconstitution be careful to read the correct set for the solution you are preparing

■ if the label does not contain reconstitution directions these may be found on the vial package insert

■ the person who reconstitutes a powdered drug must initial the vial, and print the expiration date on the label unless all the drug is used immediately

■ if a multiple strength solution is used the strength of the reconstituted drug must be printed on the label

---

SUMMARY SELF TEST

Reconstitution of Powdered Drugs

DIRECTIONS Locate the appropriate labels and answer the questions on reconstitution pertaining to them.

PART I

1. What volume of diluent must be used to reconstitute the 1 g vial of nafcillin sodium? _____

2. What will be the dosage strength of this reconstituted nafcillin? _____

3. What volume of solution must be used to reconstitute the cefazolin (Kefzol®) 250 mg vial? _____

4. What type of diluent may be used for this reconstitution? _____

5. What volume of diluent must be added to reconstitute the ampicillin 1 g vial?

   _____

6. What will the dosage strength of the prepared ampicillin solution be?

   _____

7. How long will this ampicillin solution retain its potency? _____

8. What volume of diluent is necessary to reconstitute the methicillin 6 g vial?

   _____

9. What is the dosage strength of the reconstituted solution of methicillin?

   _____

10. If this preparation is reconstituted at 3 p.m. on June 1st and stored at room temperature what expiration time and date will you print on the label?

_____

11. An IV dosage of cephapirin (Cefadyl®) 1 g in 25 mL has been ordered. What volume of diluent must you add to prepare this solution? _____

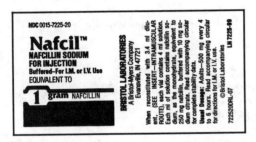

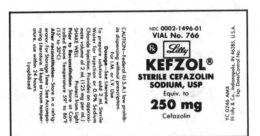

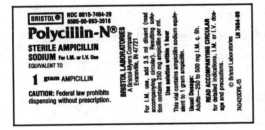

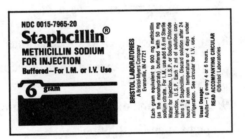

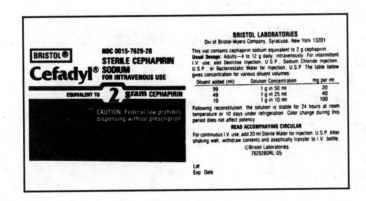

PART II

12. What volume of diluent must be used to reconstitute the methylprednisolone 500 mg vial? _____

13. What will be the dosage strength of this reconstituted methylprednisolone solution? _____

14. If a dosage of 125 mg of methylprednisolone is ordered how much solution will you prepare? _____

15. How long will the reconstituted solution of methylprednisolone retain its potency at room temperature? _____

16. What volume of diluent must be added to the 5,000,000 u vial of penicillin G to reconstitute it to a strength of 500,000 u per mL? _____

17. If a dosage of 250,000 u of penicillin G is ordered q.i.d. what would be the best strength to reconstitute, and how many mL of diluent would this require?

    _____

18. If this penicillin G was reconstituted at 6 p.m. on April 23rd and stored in the re-frigerator, what expiration date would you print on the label? _____

19. What volume of sterile water must be added to the cefuroxime 1.5 g vial to prepare an IV solution? _____

20. What volume of diluent must be added to the ceftazidime 500 mg vial for IM reconstitution? _____

21. What will the dosage strength of this reconstituted ceftazidime solution be?

    _____

22. If a dosage of ceftazidime 140 mg is ordered what volume will you draw up to prepare it? _____

NDC 0173-0354-35

Glaxo

Zinacef®
(sterile cefuroxime sodium)

1.5 g

Equivalent to 1.5 g Cefuroxime Activity.
For IV Use.

Caution: Federal law prohibits dispensing
without prescription.

See package insert for Dosage and Administration.

Store between 15° and 30°C (59° and 86°F). Protect from
light.

To prepare IV solution, add 16 ml Sterile Water for Injection.
Shake until dissolved and withdraw completely for injection.

After constitution, the solution maintains potency for 24
hours at room temperature or 48 hours under refrigeration
(5°C). Color changes in solution do not affect potency.

Glaxo Inc.,
Research Triangle Park, NC 27709
Manufactured in England
6/88

400104

NDC 0002-7230-01
VIAL No. 7230

℞ *Lilly*

TAZIDIME®
CEFTAZIDIME
FOR INJECTION

Equivalent to

500 mg

Ceftazidime Activity

For I.M. or I.V. Use

CAUTION: Addition of diluent generates pressure within the vial. Vent slowly.
For I.V. solution—Dilute with at least 5 mL Sterile Water for Injection or other approved diluent. SHAKE WELL TO DISSOLVE. See
literature.
For I.M. solution—Add 1.5 mL of an approved
diluent. SHAKE WELL TO DISSOLVE. See
literature.

Store at 59° to 86°F.
Prior to Reconstitution Protect from light.
After Reconstitution: Store in a refrigerator or use within 10 days. If kept at room
temperature, use within 24 hours. Once reconstituted, light protection is not needed.

Each vial contains 500mg of Ceftazidime and
59 mg of Sodium Carbonate. Sodium content is
approximately 27 mg (1.2 mEq) of sodium per

WW 4020 AMX
Eli Lilly & Co.,
Indianapolis, IN 46285, U.S.A.
Exp.   Date/Control No.

SQUIBB® MARSAM™

1 box • 10 vials   NDC 0003-0673-71

5,000,000 units per vial
PENICILLIN G POTASSIUM
for INJECTION USP

Caution: Federal law prohibits
dispensing without prescription

PENICILLIN G POTASSIUM for INJECTION USP

Each vial provides 5,000,000 units penicillin G potassium with approx.
135 mg citrate buffer composed of sodium citrate and not more than
4.7 mg citric acid. One million units penicillin contains approx. 1.7 mEq
potassium and 0.3 mEq sodium.

Sterile • For intramuscular or intravenous drip use
Usual dosage: See insert

PREPARATION OF SOLUTION: Add 23 mL, 18 mL, 8 mL, or 3 mL diluent
to provide 200,000 u, 250,000 u, 500,000 u, or 1,000,000 u per mL,
respectively.

Sterile solution may be kept in refrigerator 1 week without significant
loss of potency.

Store at room temperature prior to constitution
© 1986 Squibb-Marsam, Inc.

For information contact:
Squibb-Marsam, Inc., Cherry Hill, NJ 08034
Mfd. by Pfizer Inc., New York, NY 10017 Dist. by
E. R. Squibb & Sons, Inc., Princeton, NJ 08540
Made in USA   Filled in Italy   C5270 / 67371

NDC 0009-0758-01
4—125 mg doses

Solu-Medrol®
Sterile Powder
methylprednisolone sodium
succinate for injection, USP

500 mg*

For intramuscular or intravenous use

Caution: Federal law prohibits
dispensing without prescription.

Upjohn

See package insert for complete
product information

Store at controlled room temperature
15°-30° C (59°-86° F)

Reconstitute with 8.0 ml Bacteriostatic
Water for Injection with Benzyl Alcohol.
When reconstituted as directed each
8.0 ml contains *methylprednisolone
sodium succinate equivalent to 500 mg
methylprednisolone (62.5 mg per ml).

Store solution at controlled room
temperature 15°-30° C (59°-86° F)
and use within 48 hours after mixing.

Lyophilized in container

Reconstituted _____

812 365 301

The Upjohn Company
Kalamazoo, MI 49001, USA

PART III

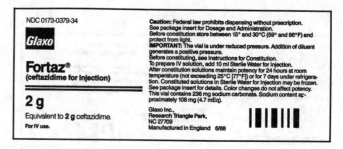

23. What volume of diluent must be used to reconstitute the 3.1 g vial of ticarcillin?

_____

24. What will be the dosage strength of this reconstituted solution? _____

25. If this ticarcillin solution is reconstituted at 8:30 a.m. on Nov 30th and stored at room temperature what expiration time and date will you print on the label?

_____

26. What volume of diluent is necessary to reconstitute the 2 g vial of ceftazidime for IV use? _____

27. What type of diluent may be used? _____

28. How long will this solution retain its potency at room temperature after reconstitution? _____

29. If the vial is reconstituted at 9 a.m. on Aug 2nd and kept under refrigeration what expiration date and time will you use to label the vial? _____

30. This label does not contain a reconstituted solution dosage strength. Where can you locate this information? _____

ANSWERS

1. 3.4 mL   2. 250 mg/mL   3. 2 mL   4. sterile water, 0.9% NaCl   5. 3.5 mL   6. 250 mg/mL   7. 1 hour   8. 8.6 mL
9. 1 g/2 mL   10. Expires 3 p.m. June 2nd   11. 49 mL   12. 8 mL   13. 62.5 mg/mL   14. 2 mL   15. 48 hours   16. 8 mL
17. 250,000 u/mL; 18 mL   18. 6 p.m. April 30th   19. 16 mL   20. 1.5 mL   21. 280 mg/mL   22. 0.5 mL   23. 13 mL
24. 200 mg/mL   25. Expires 2:30 p.m. Nov 30th   26. 10 mL   27. sterile water   28. 24 hours   29. 9 a.m. Aug 9th   30. From the package insert

SECTION
FOUR

Calculating Medication Dosages

13
Dosage Calculation Using Ratio and Proportion

OBJECTIVES
The student will use ratio and proportion to solve dosage problems containing
1. metric weights and decimal fractions
2. apothecary weights and common fractions

INTRODUCTION
In an earlier chapter you were given a thorough review of the math of ratio and proportion, and an introduction to its use in dosages. In this chapter we will concentrate on the use of ratio and proportion to solve dosage problems in the metric system, which uses decimal fractions, and in the apothecaries' system, which uses common fractions. There are three basic rules which govern all calculations: 1. routinely double check all math; 2. assess each answer obtained to determine if it is logical; and, 3. seek help if you have any question of your accuracy. Let's begin with the use of ratio and proportion for problems involving metric dosages.

• METRIC DOSAGE CALCULATIONS •

It is easier and safer to solve dosage problems if you learn to be consistent in the way you set the proportion up. A good way to do this is to **write the complete or known ratio first**. This will always be the dosage strength of the drug available which you will read from the drug label. **The incomplete or unknown ratio is the dosage ordered, and it is written second.** Let's look at some examples.

EXAMPLE 1   Order: Administer 700 mg of a drug which has a dosage strength of 500 mg per 2 mL. Express your answer to the nearest tenth.

500 mg : 2 mL = 700 mg : X mL

$\left(\begin{array}{cc}\text{complete ratio} & \text{incomplete ratio} \\ \text{drug strength} & \text{dosage ordered}\end{array}\right)$

Do not forget the critical step of **writing the ratios in the same sequence of measurement units**. In the example above this was done; **mg : mL = mg : mL** With the proportion correctly set up the math is exactly as you have practiced: multiply the means and the extremes and divide by the number in front of X.

500 mg : 2 mL = 700 mg : X mL

$2 \times 700 = 500X$

$$\frac{2 \times 700}{500} = X = \textbf{2.8 mL}$$

After you have double checked your math assess the answer to determine if it is logical. If 500 mg equals 2 mL it will require more then 2 mL to obtain a dosage of 700 mg. Your answer, 2.8 mL is larger, therefore it is logical. This routine check does not prove that your math is correct, but it does indicate that you have not mixed up the means and extremes in your calculations.

EXAMPLE 2   A drug label reads 100 mg per 2 mL. The medication order is for 130 mg. How many mL must you administer?

$$100 \text{ mg} : 2 \text{ mL} = 130 \text{ mg} : X \text{ mL}$$

$$2 \times 130 = 100X$$

$$\frac{2 \times 130}{100} = X = \textbf{2.6 mL}$$

130 mg is a larger dosage than the 100 mg per 2 mL available, and must be contained in a larger volume. Your answer, 2.6 mL, is a larger volume.

EXAMPLE 3:   The order is to give 0.15 g of medication. The dosage strength available is 200 mg/mL.

This problem cannot be solved as it is now written because the drug weights are in different units of measure: g and mg. In a previous chapter you learned that it is safer to convert down the scale, higher units to lower, to eliminate or avoid decimals. Convert the g to mg.

$$200 \text{ mg} : 1 \text{ mL} = 0.15 \text{ g} : X \text{ mL}$$

Convert g to mg

$$200 \text{ mg} : 1 \text{ mL} = 150 \text{ mg} : X \text{ mL}$$

$$1 \times 150 = 200X$$

$$\frac{150}{200} = X = 0.75 = \textbf{0.8 mL}$$

EXAMPLE 4   Ratio and proportion can also be used to solve dosage calculations for measures other than metric, for example international units. The order is to give 1200 u. The available dosage strength is 1000 u per 1.5 mL.

$$1000 \text{ u} : 1.5 \text{ mL} = 1200 \text{ u} : X \text{ mL}$$

$$1.5 \times 1200 = 1000X$$

$$\frac{1.5 \times 1200}{1000} = X = \textbf{1.8 mL}$$

PROBLEM

Solve the following dosage problems. Express answers to the nearest tenth.

1. The drug label reads 1000 mcg in 2 mL. The order is 0.4 mg.

2. The ordered dosage is 275 mg. The available drug is labeled 0.5 g per 2 mL.

3. A dosage strength of 0.2 mg in 1.5 mL is available. Give 0.15 mg.

4. The strength available is 1 g in 3.6 mL. Prepare a 600 mg dosage.

5. A 10,000 u dosage has been ordered. The dosage strength available is 8,000 u in 1 mL.

ANSWERS   **1.** 0.8 mL **2.** 1.1 mL **3.** 1.1 mL **4.** 2.2 mL **5.** 1.3 mL

• APOTHECARY DOSAGE CALCULATIONS •

Calculations in apothecary measures are set up the same as for metric calculations. The dosage available will provide the complete or known ratio. The dosage to be given will provide the incomplete ratio.

EXAMPLE 1   The drug available has a strength of gr $\frac{1}{150}$ in 1 mL. You must administer gr $\frac{1}{100}$.

$$\text{gr}\,\frac{1}{150} : 1\ \text{mL} = \text{gr}\,\frac{1}{100} : X\ \text{mL}$$

$$1 \times \frac{1}{100} = \frac{1}{150}X$$

$$\frac{\dfrac{1}{100}}{\dfrac{1}{150}} = X$$

$$\frac{1}{100} \times \frac{150}{1} = X = \textbf{1.5 mL}$$

gr $\frac{1}{100}$ is a larger dosage than gr $\frac{1}{150}$ and must be contained in a larger volume than 1 mL.

EXAMPLE 2   Drug strength is gr $\frac{1}{8}$ in 1.5 mL. Prepare a gr $\frac{1}{6}$ dosage.

$$\text{gr}\,\frac{1}{8} : 1.5\ \text{mL} = \text{gr}\,\frac{1}{6} : X\ \text{mL}$$

$$1.5 \times \frac{1}{6} = \frac{1}{8}X$$

$$\frac{1.5 \times \dfrac{1}{6}}{\dfrac{1}{8}} = X$$

$$1.5 \times \frac{1}{6} \times \frac{8}{1} = X = \textbf{2 mL}$$

To administer a dosage of gr $\frac{1}{6}$ you must give 2 mL.

EXAMPLE 3   A drug is labeled gr ½ per 2 mL. Prepare a gr ⅓ dosage.

$$\text{gr } \frac{1}{2} : 2 \text{ mL} = \text{gr } \frac{1}{3} : X \text{ mL}$$

$$2 \times \frac{1}{3} = \frac{1}{2}X$$

$$\frac{2 \times \frac{1}{3}}{\frac{1}{2}} = X$$

$$2 \times \frac{1}{3} \times \frac{2}{1} = X = \textbf{1.3 mL}$$

PROBLEM

Calculate the dosage in mL which must be administered in the following problems. Express answers to the nearest tenth.

1. Prepare a gr ¹⁄₂₀₀ dosage of solution from an available strength of gr ¹⁄₁₅₀ in 2.5 mL.

2. The drug strength is gr ¼ in 2 mL. Prepare gr ⅙.

3. A dosage of gr ⅙ has been ordered. The strength available is gr ¼ in 1.2 mL.

4. A dosage strength of gr ¹⁄₁₀₀ per 1 mL is available. A dosage of gr ¹⁄₅₀ has been ordered.

5. A dosage of gr ¹⁄₇₅ has been ordered. The strength available is gr ¹⁄₅₀ in 2 mL.

ANSWERS   **1.** 1.9 mL   **2.** 1.3 mL   **3.** 0.8 mL   **4.** 2 mL   **5.** 1.3 mL

This concludes the chapter on dosage calculations. The important points to remember from this chapter are:

■ the available dosage strength provides the complete or known ratio for calculations

■ the dosage to be given provides the incomplete or unknown ratio

■ the ratios in a proportion must be set up in the same sequence of measurement units, for example mg : mL = mg : mL

■ if the measurement units in a calculation are different, for example mg and g, one of these must be converted before the problem can be solved

■ the math of all calculations is routinely double checked

■ a logical assessment of the answer you obtain is a routine step in your calculations

■ if you have any doubt of your accuracy in calculations seek help

Dosage Calculation Using Ratio and Proportion

DIRECTIONS Read the medication labels provided and calculate the volume necessary to provide the dosage ordered. Express your answers as decimal fractions to the nearest tenth, unless instructed otherwise.

PART I

1. Prepare a dosage of 20 mg of Zantac® _____

2. Prepare a 300 mcg dosage of naloxone _____

3. Prepare a 50 mg dosage of gentamicin _____

4. Furosemide 15 mg has been ordered _____

5. A dosage of perphenazine 7 mg is ordered _____

6. The order is for 70 mg of tobramycin _____

7. An order reads: dexamethasone 5 mg _____

8. Draw up 30 mEq of sodium bicarbonate _____

9. Prepare nitroglycerine 12 mg _____

10. The dosage is Depo-Provera® 140 mg _____

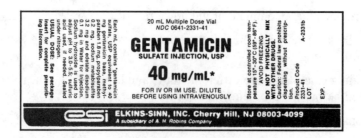

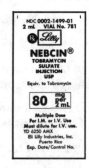

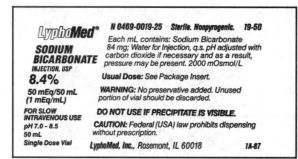

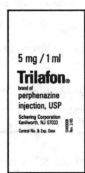

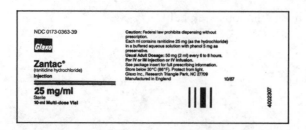

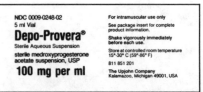

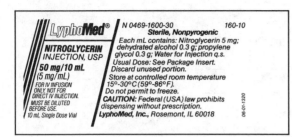

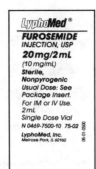

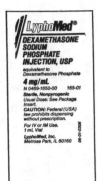

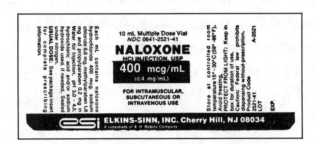

PART II

11. Draw up 7,500 u of heparin. Calculate dosage to hundredths _____

12. Lincocin® 350 mg has been ordered _____

13. Draw up a 400 mg dosage of aminophylline _____

14. Prepare a 170 mg dosage of amikacin _____

15. Morphine gr ⅙ has been ordered _____

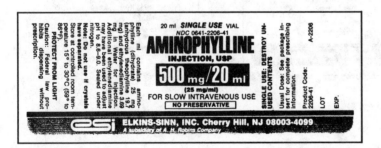

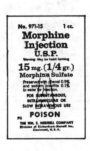

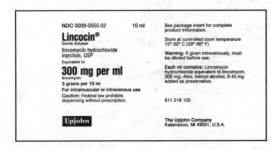

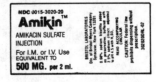

PART III

16. Prepare 80 mg meperidine for IM injection _____

17. Atropine 0.2 mg has been ordered _____

18. Tigan® 250 mg has been ordered _____

19. Garamycin® 100 mg has been ordered _____

20. Kanamycin 800 mg has been ordered _____

21. Prepare cyanocobalamin 1500 mcg _____

22. Draw up 50 mg of tobramycin _____

23. A dosage of Pronestyl® 600 mg is to be prepared _____

24. Prepare a 400,000 u dosage of Duracillin® AS _____

25. Measure 650 u of heparin to the nearest hundredth _____

26. Prepare a 5 mg dosage of Celestone® _____

27. Prepare a gr ½ dosage of Seconal® _____

28. Prepare an 8 mg dosage of morphine _____

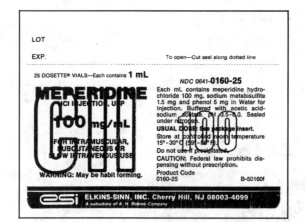

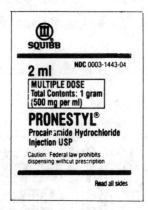

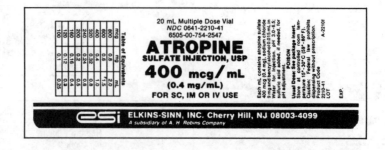

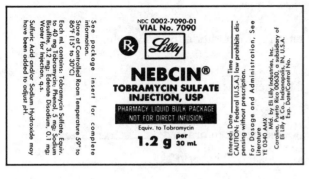

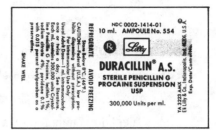

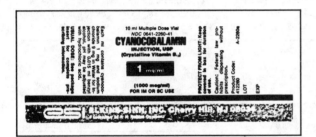

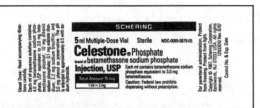

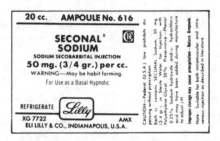

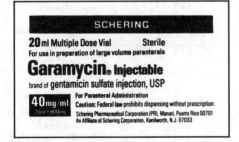

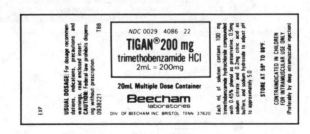

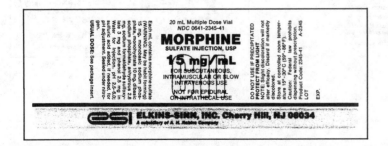

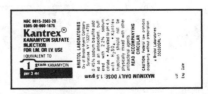

PART IV

29. Prepare 20 mEq of potassium chloride for addition to an IV solution

   _____

30. A dosage of diazepam 7.5 mg has been ordered _____

31. Prepare an 8 mg dosage of Trandate® _____

32. An 80 mg dosage of dromostanolone has been ordered _____

33. Calculate to hundredths a 4,500 u dosage of heparin _____

34. Measure a 16 mg dosage of Aramine® _____

35. Atropine gr ¹⁄₁₀₀ has been ordered _____

36. Measure a 450 mg dosage of Depo-Provera® _____

37. Compazine® 8 mg has been ordered _____

38. Prepare a 90 mg dosage of phenytoin _____

39. Give Vistaril® 70 mg IM _____

40. Measure a 275 mg dosage of clindamycin _____

ANSWERS

1. 0.8 mL   2. 0.8 mL   3. 1.3 mL   4. 1.5 mL   5. 1.4 mL   6. 1.8 mL   7. 1.3 mL   8. 30 mL   9. 2.4 mL   10. 1.4 mL
11. 0.75 mL   12. 1.2 mL   13. 16 mL   14. 0.7 mL   15. 0.7 cc   16. 0.8 mL   17. 0.5 mL   18. 2.5 mL   19. 2.5 mL   20. 2.4 mL
21. 1.5 mL   22. 1.3 mL   23. 1.2 mL   24. 1.3 mL   25. 0.65 mL   26. 1.7 mL   27. 0.7 mL   28. 0.5 mL   29. 10 mL   30. 1.5 mL
31. 1.6 mL   32. 1.6 mL   33. 0.9 mL   34. 1.6 mL   35. 1.5 mL   36. 1.1 mL   37. 1.6 mL   38. 1.8 mL   39. 1.4 cc   40. 1.8 mL

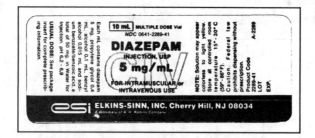

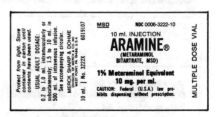

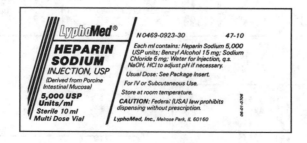

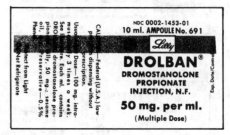

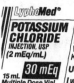

LyphoMed®
POTASSIUM CHLORIDE
INJECTION, USP
(2 mEq/mL)

15 mL
Multiple Dose Vial

30 mEq

N 0469-1567-15 Sterile. Nonpyrogenic. 967-15
MUST BE DILUTED PRIOR TO IV ADMINISTRATION
Each mL contains: Potassium Chloride 149 mg;
Methylparaben 0.05%; Propylparaben 0.005%;
Water for Injection q.s. pH adjusted with HCl or
KOH if necessary. 4000 mOsmol/L.
Usual Dose: See Package Insert.
LyphoMed, Inc., Rosemont, IL 60018   B-87

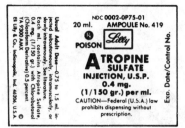

NDC 0002-0P75-01
20 ml.   AMPOULE No. 419
℞ *Lilly*
POISON
ATROPINE SULFATE
INJECTION, U.S.P.
0.4 mg.
(1/150 gr.) per ml.
CAUTION—Federal (U.S.A.) law
prohibits dispensing without
prescription.

Usual Adult Dose—0.75 to 1.5 ml. in-
jected subcutaneously, intramuscularly, or
slowly intravenously. See literature.
Each ml. contains Atropine Sulfate,
0.4 mg. (1/150 gr.) with Chlorobutanol
(Chloroform Derivative) 0.5 percent.
YA 9300 AMX
Eli Lilly & Co., Indianapolis, Ind. 46206, U.S.A.

Exp. Date/Control No.

NDC 0009-0728-05
6505-01-246-8718

60 ml Pharmacy
Bulk Package

Not for direct infusion
Cleocin Phosphate®
Sterile Solution
clindamycin phosphate injection, USP
Equivalent to clindamycin

150 mg per ml

For intramuscular or intravenous use
Caution: Federal law prohibits
dispensing without prescription.

Upjohn The Upjohn Company
Kalamazoo, MI 49001, USA

LyphoMed®
PHENYTOIN SODIUM
INJECTION, USP
250 mg (50 mg/mL)
**FOR IV (Not Infusion)
OR IM USE**
5 mL
SINGLE DOSE VIAL

N 0469-1615-25 Sterile. No. 615-05
Each mL contains: Phenytoin
Sodium 50 mg; Propylene Glycol
0.4 mL; Alcohol 0.1 mL; Water
for Injection, q.s. pH adjusted
with NaOH, if necessary.
Discard unused portion.
Usual Dose: See Insert.
WARNING: Do not use the injection
if it is hazy or contains a precipitate.
LyphoMed, Inc., Rosemont, IL 60018 K-86

NDC 0173-0350-58

Glaxo

Trandate®
(labetalol hydrochloride)
Injection

5 mg/ml
(100 mg in 20 ml)
For IV Injection only.
20 ml Multi-dose Vial   **Sterile**

Caution: Federal law prohibits dispensing without prescription.
See package insert for Dosage and Administration.
Store between 2° and 30°C (36° and 86°F). Do not freeze.
Protect from light.
Each 1 ml of aqueous solution contains labetalol hydrochloride
5 mg; anhydrous dextrose 45 mg; edetate disodium 0.1 mg;
citric acid monohydrate and sodium hydroxide as necessary to
bring the pH into range; methylparaben 0.8 mg and
propylparaben 0.1 mg as preservatives.
Glaxo Inc.,
Research Triangle Park, NC 27709
Manufactured in England
2/88

4004625

---

2 cc.
Vistaril®
hydroxyzine
hydrochloride
INTRAMUSCULAR SOLUTION
100 mg./2 cc.
FOR IM USE ONLY
Pfizer LABORATORIES
DIVISION
PFIZER INC.

NDC 0007-0C43-01

Keep in a cool place, but avoid freezing
PROTECT FROM LIGHT

Each ml. contains, in aqueous solution, prochlorperazine, 5 mg., as the edisylate; sodium
biphosphate, 5 mg.; sodium tartrate, 12 mg.;
sodium saccharin, 0.9 mg. Contains benzyl
alcohol, 0.75%, as preservative.

See accompanying folder for complete prescribing data.
          Patent 2902484

for deep IM or IV injection
Compazine® 10 ml.
brand of
prochlorperazine Multiple-
dose Vial
Injection 5 mg./ml.
CAUTION—Federal law prohibits
dispensing without prescription.
Smith Kline & French Laboratories
Div. of SmithKline Corp.
Phila., Pa. 19101

NDC 0009-0626-01
2.5 ml Vial
Depo-Provera®
Sterile Aqueous Suspension
sterile medroxyprogesterone
acetate suspension, USP
400 mg per ml

For IM use only
See package insert for complete
product information.
Shake vigorously immediately
before each use.
812 224 201
The Upjohn Company
Kalamazoo, Michigan 49001, USA

14
Dosage Calculation Using the Formula Method

OBJECTIVES

The student will use a formula to solve dosage problems containing
1. metric weights and decimal fractions
2. apothecary weights and common fractions

INTRODUCTION

This chapter will teach you how to use a simple formula for ratio and proportion to set up and solve dosage problems. All the math necessary to use the formula method has been covered in previous chapters, and will be familiar to you. The formula is as follows:

FORMULA

$$\frac{D}{H} \times Q = X$$

Here is what these initials mean.

D = **desired.** The dosage ordered, in mg, g, etc.
H = **have.** The dosage strength available, in mg, g, etc.
Q = **quantity.** The volume the dosage strength available is contained in, mL, cc, etc.
X = **the unknown.** The volume the desired dosage will be contained in.

   It is necessary to memorize this formula. Stop and do so now. Print the formula several times to help yourself remember it.
   There are three guidelines or rules which govern all calculations. These are: 1. routinely double check all math; 2. assess each answer to determine if it is logical; and, 3. seek help if you have any doubt of your accuracy. Let's begin by looking at the use of the formula in metric calculations.

• METRIC DOSAGE CALCULATION •

Here are some sample dosage problems which contain metric measures.

EXAMPLE 1   A dosage of 80 mg is ordered. The dosage strength available is 100 mg in 2 mL. The desired (D) is 80 mg. You have (H) 100 mg in (Q) 2 mL. X will always be expressed in the same units of measure as the Q, in this problem, mL. Always set up the formula with the units of measure included.

$$\frac{(D)\ 80\ mg}{(H)\ 100\ mg} \times (Q)\ 2\ mL = X\ mL$$

$$\frac{80}{100} \times 2 = X = \mathbf{1.6\ mL}$$

To give a dosage of 80 mg you must administer 1.6 mL. After you have double checked your math look at your answer to see if it is logical. The dosage strength available is 100 mg in 2 mL. To prepare 80 mg, which is a smaller dosage, you will need a smaller volume. Your answer, 1.6 mL, is smaller therefore it is logical. This check does not guarantee that your math is correct, but it does indicate that you have correctly placed the dosages in the formula.

EXAMPLE 2   The dosage ordered is 0.4 mg. The strength available is 0.25 mg in 1.2 mL.

$$\frac{0.4\ mg}{0.25\ mg} \times 1.2\ mL = X\ mL = \mathbf{1.9\ mL}$$

0.4 mg is a larger dosage than 0.25 mg and the volume which contains it must be larger, which it is: 1.9 mL.

EXAMPLE 3   A dosage of 200 mcg is ordered. The strength available is 0.3 mg in 1.5 mL.

This problem cannot be solved as it is now written. **D and H, the drug strengths, must be expressed in the same units of measure.** As in earlier chapters where you practiced conversions it may be somewhat less confusing to change the higher unit to a lower one, for example, the 0.3 **mg** to **mcg**, in order to eliminate a decimal point.

0.3 mg = 300 mcg

$$\frac{200\ mcg}{300\ mcg} \times 1.5\ mL = X\ mL = \mathbf{1\ mL}$$

To administer 200 mcg you must give 1 mL of the 0.3 mg in 1.5 mL dosage strength.

The formula may also be used to solve dosages expressed in measures other than metric, for example international units.

EXAMPLE 4   A dosage of 7500 u is ordered. The available strength is 10,000 u per mL.

$$\frac{7500\ u}{10,000\ u} \times 1\ mL = X\ mL = 0.75 = \mathbf{0.8\ mL}$$

Determine the volume which will contain the dosage ordered in the following problems. Express answers as decimal fractions to the nearest tenth.

1. The dosage ordered is 780 mcg. The strength available is 1 mg per mL.

_____

2. A dosage of 0.8 g has been ordered. The strength available is 1 g in 2.5 mL.

_____

3. The available dosage strength is 0.1 g per mL. The dosage ordered is 250 mg.

_____

4. A dosage strength of 1000 u per 1.5 mL is available. Prepare a 1250 u dosage.

_____

5. Prepare a dosage of 0.4 mg from an available strength of 1000 mcg per 2 mL.

_____

ANSWERS   **1.** 0.8 mL   **2.** 2 mL   **3.** 2.5 mL   **4.** 1.9 mL   **5.** 0.8 mL

• APOTHECARY DOSAGE CALCULATIONS •

Apothecary dosages expressed as common fractions are also solved using the formula method.

EXAMPLE 1   The dosage available is gr ¼ in 1 mL. Prepare gr ⅙.

$$\frac{gr \dfrac{1}{6}}{gr \dfrac{1}{4}} \times 1 \text{ mL} = X \text{ mL}$$

$$\frac{1}{6} \times \frac{4}{1} = X = 0.66 = \textbf{0.7 mL}$$

gr ⅙ is a smaller dosage than gr ¼ and it is contained in a smaller volume, 0.7 mL.

EXAMPLE 2   A solution is labeled gr ¹⁄₁₅₀ in 1.5 mL. Give gr ¹⁄₂₀₀.

$$\frac{gr \dfrac{1}{200}}{gr \dfrac{1}{150}} \times 1.5 \text{ mL} = X \text{ mL}$$

$$\frac{1}{200} \times \frac{150}{1} \times 1.5 = X = \mathbf{1.1\ mL}$$

EXAMPLE 3 The dosage strength is gr 1/8 in 1 mL. Prepare gr 1/10.

$$\frac{\text{gr}\ \frac{1}{10}}{\text{gr}\ \frac{1}{8}} \times 1\ \text{mL} = X\ \text{mL}$$

$$\frac{1}{10} \times \frac{8}{1} \times 1 = X = \mathbf{0.8\ mL}$$

PROBLEM

In the following problems calculate in mL the dosages ordered. Express answers to the nearest tenth.

1. A drug is labeled gr 1/2 in 2 mL. Prepare gr 1/4 ____________

2. The order is for gr 1/8. The strength available is gr 1/6 in 1.5 mL ____________

3. A dosage of gr 1/150 is ordered. The strength available is gr 1/100 in 2 mL

   ____

4. A dosage of gr 1/8 in 1 mL is available; gr 1/6 is ordered ____________

5. Prepare a dosage of gr 1/4 from an available strength of gr 1/2 in 1.5 mL

   ____

ANSWERS **1.** 1 mL **2.** 1.1 mL **3.** 1.3 mL **4.** 1.3 mL **5.** 0.8 mL

This concludes the chapter on using the formula method to solve dosage calculations. The important points to remember from this chapter are:

- the formula method can be used to solve problems expressed in metric, apothecary, and other measures such as international units
- D = desired; H = have; Q = quantity; X = the unknown
- when the formula method is used, D and H, the dosage strengths, must be expressed in the same units of measure
- the math of all calculations is routinely double checked
- a logical assessment of the answer you obtain is a routine step in calculations

---

SUMMARY SELF TEST

Dosage Calculation Using the Formula Method

DIRECTIONS Read the labels provided to calculate the dosages ordered in the following problems. Express your answers as decimal fractions to the nearest tenth unless instructed otherwise.

PART I

1. A 50 mg dosage of gentamicin has been ordered _____

2. Prepare a 300 mcg dosage of atropine. Calculate to the nearest hundredth _____

3. Prepare lincomycin 0.45 g _____

4. Diazepam 8 mg has been ordered _____

5. Prepare a 70 mg dosage of phenytoin _____

6. Vistaril® 30 mg has been ordered _____

7. Prepare a 60 mg dosage of meperidine _____

8. The order is for Compazine® 12 mg _____

9. Dolophine® 7 mg has been ordered _____

10. Morphine 8 mg has been ordered _____

11. Prepare a 0.3 g dosage of clindamycin _____

12. Prepare a 300 mg dosage of aminophylline _____

13. A dosage of kanamycin 750 mg has been ordered _____

14. Prepare a dosage of fentanyl 0.2 mg _____

15. The order is for amikacin 130 mg _____

SCHERING

Garamycin® INJECTABLE   NDC-0085-0069-05   **60 mg**
brand of   1.5ml = 60mg
gentamicin sulfate injection, USP

Each ml contains gentamicin sulfate,
USP equivalent to 40 mg gentamicin.

Caution: Federal law prohibits dispensing without prescription.

LyphoMed® N 0469-1615-25 Sterile. No. 615-05
PHENYTOIN SODIUM INJECTION, USP
Each mL contains: Phenytoin Sodium 50 mg; Propylene Glycol 0.4 mL; Alcohol 0.1 mL; Water for Injection, q.s. pH adjusted with NaOH, if necessary.
250 mg (50 mg/mL)
FOR IV (Not Infusion) OR IM USE
5 mL
SINGLE DOSE VIAL
Discard unused portion.
Usual Dose: See Insert.
WARNING: Do not use the injection if it is hazy or contains a precipitate. LyphoMed. inc., Rosemont, IL 60018 K-86

NDC 0009-3447-01   Single Dose
6 ml ADD-Vantage™ Vial

Cleocin Phosphate®
Sterile Solution
clindamycin phosphate
injection, USP

900 mg

Equivalent to 900 mg clindamycin

Use only with the ADD-Vantage diluent container.
See package insert for complete product information.
Store at controlled room temperature 15°-30° C (59°-86° F)
™Trademark of Abbott Laboratories
813 897 000

The Upjohn Company
Kalamazoo, MI 49001, USA

Upjohn

900 mg
Cleocin Phosphate®
clindamycin phosphate Injection, USP

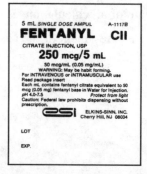

5 mL SINGLE DOSE AMPUL   A-1117B
FENTANYL   CII
CITRATE INJECTION, USP
250 mcg/5 mL
50 mcg/mL (0.05 mg/mL)
WARNING: May be habit forming.
For INTRAVENOUS or INTRAMUSCULAR use
Read package insert
Each mL contains fentanyl citrate equivalent to 50 mcg (0.05 mg) fentanyl base in Water for Injection.
pH 4.0-7.5   Protect from light
Caution: Federal law prohibits dispensing without prescription.

ELKINS-SINN, INC.
Cherry Hill, NJ 08034

LOT

EXP.

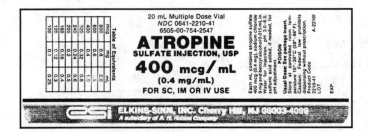

20 mL Multiple Dose Vial
NDC 0641-2210-41
6505-00-754-2547

ATROPINE
SULFATE INJECTION, USP
400 mcg/mL
(0.4 mg/mL)
FOR SC, IM OR IV USE

Each mL contains atropine sulfate
400 mcg (0.4 mg), sodium chloride
9 mg and benzyl alcohol 0.015 mL in
Water for Injection. pH 3.0-6.5;
sulfuric acid added, if needed, for
pH adjustment. POISON
Usual Dose: See package insert.
Store at controlled room temperature 15°-30°C (59°-86° F).
Caution: Federal law prohibits
dispensing without prescription.
Product Code
2210-41
LOT
EXP.   A-2210f

eSi ELKINS-SINN, INC. Cherry Hill, NJ 08003-4099
A subsidiary of A. H. Robins Company

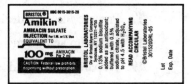

BRISTOL · NDC 0015-3015-20
Amikin®
AMIKACIN SULFATE
INJECTION For I.M. or I.V. Use
EQUIVALENT TO
100 mg AMIKACIN
Per 2 ml

BRISTOL LABORATORIES
Div. of Bristol-Myers Company
Syracuse, NY 13221-4755
0.13% sodium bisulfite
added as an antioxidant;
buffered with 0.5%
sodium citrate, adjusted
to pH 4.5 with H_2SO_4.
READ ACCOMPANYING
CIRCULAR
©Bristol Laboratories
3015200RL-05
Lot
Exp. Date

CAUTION: Federal law prohibits
dispensing without prescription.

LOT

EXP.   To open—Cut seal along dotted line

25 DOSETTE® AMPULS   Each contains **1 mL**
NDC 0641-**1130-35**

MEPERIDINE
HCl INJECTION, USP
50 mg/mL

**FOR INTRAMUSCULAR, SUBCUTANEOUS OR
SLOW INTRAVENOUS USE**

Warning: May be habit forming.
Each mL contains meperidine hydrochloride 50 mg in Water for
Injection. pH 3.5-6.0; sodium hydroxide and/or hydrochloric acid
added, if needed, for pH adjustment. Sealed under nitrogen.
USUAL DOSE: See package insert.
DO NOT USE IF PRECIPITATED.
Store at controlled room temperature 15°-30°C (59°-86°F).
Caution: Federal law prohibits dispensing without prescription.
To open ampuls, ignore color line; break at constriction.
Product Code: 1130-35   B-51130d

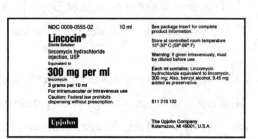

NDC 0009-0555-02   10 ml

Lincocin®
Sterile Solution
lincomycin hydrochloride
injection, USP
Equivalent to
300 mg per ml
lincomycin
3 grams per 10 ml
For intramuscular or intravenous use
Caution: Federal law prohibits
dispensing without prescription.

See package insert for complete
product information.

Store at controlled room temperature
15°-30° C (59°-86° F)

Warning: If given intravenously, must
be diluted before use.

Each ml contains: Lincomycin
hydrochloride equivalent to lincomycin,
300 mg; Also, benzyl alcohol, 9.45 mg
added as preservative.

811 218 102

Upjohn   The Upjohn Company
Kalamazoo, MI 49001, U.S.A.

NDC 0015-3502-20
Kantrex®
KANAMYCIN
SULFATE INJECTION
FOR I.M. OR I.V. USE
EQUIVALENT TO
0.5 Gm.
KANAMYCIN
per 2 ml.

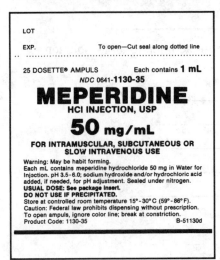

10 mL MULTIPLE DOSE Vial
NDC 0641-2343-41   A-2343s

MORPHINE
SULFATE INJECTION, USP
10 mg/1 mL
FOR SUBCUTANEOUS,
INTRAMUSCULAR OR SLOW
INTRAVENOUS USE
NOT FOR EPIDURAL
OR INTRATHECAL USE

Each mL contains morphine
sulfate (WARNING: May be habit
forming) 10 mg, dibasic sodium
phosphate 10 mg, sodium
formaldehyde sulfoxylate 3 mg and
phenol 2.5 mg in...

eSi ELKINS-SINN, INC. Cherry Hill, NJ 08034

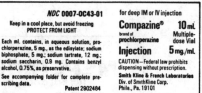

NDC 0007-0C43-01

Keep in a cool place, but avoid freezing
PROTECT FROM LIGHT

Each ml. contains, in aqueous solution, prochlorperazine, 5 mg., as the edisylate; sodium
biphosphate, 5 mg.; sodium tartrate, 12 mg.;
sodium saccharin, 0.9 mg. Contains benzyl
alcohol, 0.75%, as preservative.

See accompanying folder for complete prescribing data.   Patent 2902484

for deep IM or IV injection
Compazine®   10 ml.
brand of   Multiple-
prochlorperazine   dose Vial
Injection   5 mg./ml.

CAUTION—Federal law prohibits
dispensing without prescription.

Smith Kline & French Laboratories
Div. of SmithKline Corp.
Phila., Pa. 19101

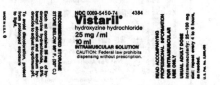

NDC 0069-5450-74   4384
Vistaril®
hydroxyzine hydrochloride
25 mg /ml
10 ml
INTRAMUSCULAR SOLUTION
CAUTION: Federal law prohibits
dispensing without prescription.

READ ACCOMPANYING
PROFESSIONAL INFORMATION
FOR INTRAMUSCULAR
USE ONLY

USUAL ADULT DOSE
Intramuscularly: 25-100 mg
IM, repeat every 4 to 6 hours.

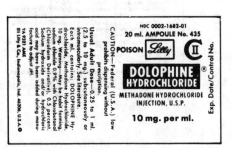

NDC 0002-1682-01
20 ml. AMPOULE No. 435
POISON Lilly CII
**DOLOPHINE®
HYDROCHLORIDE**
METHADONE HYDROCHLORIDE
INJECTION, U.S.P.
10 mg. per ml.

Usual Adult Dose—0.25 to 1 ml.
(2.5 to 10 mg.) subcutaneously or
intramuscularly. See literature.

Each ml. contains: DOLOPHINE Hydrochloride, 10 mg. (Warning—May be habit forming,
(Chloroform Derivative), 0.5 percent.
Sodium hydroxide and/or hydrochloric
acid may have been added during manufacture to adjust pH.

CAUTION—Federal law
prohibits dispensing without
prescription.

Exp. Date/Control No.

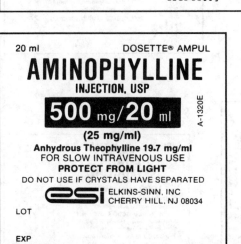

20 ml   **DOSETTE® AMPUL**

AMINOPHYLLINE
INJECTION, USP
500 mg/20 ml
(25 mg/ml)   A-1320E
Anhydrous Theophylline 19.7 mg/ml
FOR SLOW INTRAVENOUS USE
PROTECT FROM LIGHT
DO NOT USE IF CRYSTALS HAVE SEPARATED

eSi ELKINS-SINN, INC
CHERRY HILL, NJ 08034

LOT

EXP

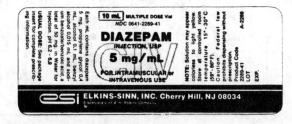

10 mL MULTIPLE DOSE Vial
NDC 0641-2289-41   A-2289

DIAZEPAM
INJECTION, USP
5 mg/mL
FOR INTRAMUSCULAR OR
INTRAVENOUS USE

Each mL contains diazepam
5 mg, propylene glycol 0.4
mL, alcohol 0.015 mL, benzyl
alcohol 0.015 mL in Water for
Injection. pH 6.2-6.9.
USUAL DOSE: See package insert.
Store at controlled room
temperature 15°-30°C
(59°-86°F).
Caution: Federal law
prohibits dispensing without
prescription.
Product Code
2289-41
LOT
EXP.

NOTE: Solution may appear
colorless to light yellow.

eSi ELKINS-SINN, INC. Cherry Hill, NJ 08034
A subsidiary of A. H. Robins Company

PART II

16. Draw up a 12 mg dosage of betamethasone _____

17. Prepare furosemide 14 mg _____

18. Draw up an 800 mg dosage of tobramycin for IV dilution _____

19. Prepare an 80 mg dosage of Trandate® _____

20. Atropine gr ⅓₀₀ is ordered _____

21. Prepare a 600 mg dosage of Depo-Provera® _____

22. Draw up an 80 mEq dosage of sodium acetate for addition to an IV solution

_____

23. Naloxone 0.6 mg has been ordered _____

24. Prepare a 60 mg dosage of meperidine _____

25. Prepare a 100 mg dosage of Garamycin® _____

26. The order is for nitroglycerin 8 mg _____

27. Measure a 0.8 mg dosage of Neo-Betalin® _____

28. Prepare Zantac® 40 mg _____

29. Dexamethasone 10 mg has been ordered _____

30. Prepare 200 mg of protamine for IV use _____

31. Morphine 10 mg has been ordered. Measure to the nearest hundredth

_____

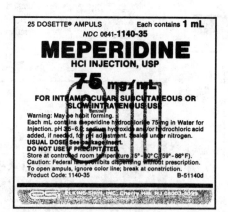

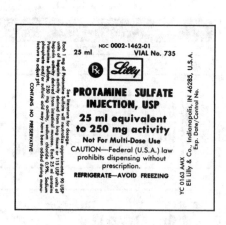

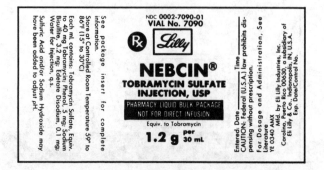

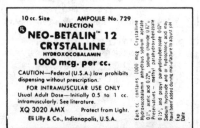

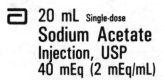

20 mL Single-dose
Sodium Acetate
Injection, USP
40 mEq (2 mEq/mL)
CAUTION: MUST BE DILUTED

ABBOTT LABORATORIES, NORTH CHICAGO, IL 60064, USA

NDC 0074-7299-01
Each mL contains sodium acetate, anhyd.
164 mg. May contain acetic acid for pH
adjustment. 4 mOsm/mL (calc.). pH 6.0 to 7.0.
Sterile, nonpyrogenic. For intravenous use.
Usual dose: See insert. Caution: Federal (USA)
law prohibits dispensing without prescription.
06-5398-2/R5-11/86

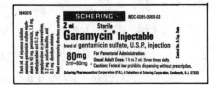

SCHERING   NDC-0085-0069-03
2 ml Sterile
Garamycin® Injectable
brand of gentamicin sulfate, U.S.P., injection
80mg
For Parenteral Administration
Usual Adult Dose: 1½ to 2 ml. three times daily.
2ml=80mg → Caution: Federal law prohibits dispensing without prescription.
Schering Pharmaceutical Corporation (P.R.), A Subsidiary of Schering Corporation, Kenilworth, N.J. 07033

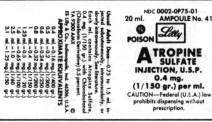

NDC 0002-0P75-01
20 mL.   AMPOULE No. 419
POISON   Lilly
ATROPINE SULFATE
INJECTION, U.S.P.
0.4 mg.
(1/150 gr.) per ml.
CAUTION—Federal (U.S.A.) law
prohibits dispensing without
prescription.

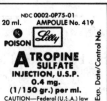

LyphoMed®
FUROSEMIDE
INJECTION, USP
20 mg/2 mL
(10 mg/mL)
Sterile,
Nonpyrogenic
Usual Dose: See
Package Insert.
For IM or IV Use.
2 mL
Single Dose Vial
N 0469-7500-10 75-02
LyphoMed, Inc.
Melrose Park, IL 60160

NDC 0009-0626-01
2.5 ml Vial   For IM use only
See package insert for complete
product information.
Depo-Provera®
Sterile Aqueous Suspension   Shake vigorously immediately
sterile medroxyprogesterone   before each use.
acetate suspension, USP
2mL
400 mg per ml   812 224 201
The Upjohn Company
Kalamazoo, Michigan 49001, USA

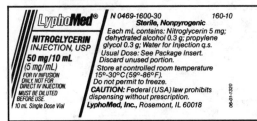

LyphoMed®
NITROGLYCERIN
INJECTION, USP
50 mg/10 mL
(5 mg/mL)
FOR IV INFUSION
ONLY. NOT FOR
DIRECT IV INJECTION.
MUST BE DILUTED
BEFORE USE.
10 mL Single Dose Vial

N 0469-1600-30   160-10
Sterile, Nonpyrogenic
Each mL contains: Nitroglycerin 5 mg;
dehydrated alcohol 0.3 g; propylene
glycol 0.3 g; Water for Injection q.s.
Usual Dose: See Package Insert.
Discard unused portion.
Store at controlled room temperature
15°-30°C (59°-86°F).
Do not permit to freeze.
CAUTION: Federal (USA) law prohibits
dispensing without prescription.
LyphoMed, Inc., Rosemont, IL 60018
06-01-1320

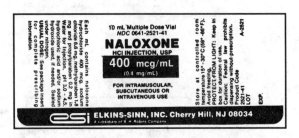

10 mL Multiple Dose Vial
NDC 0641-2521-41
NALOXONE
HCl INJECTION, USP
400 mcg/mL
(0.4 mg/mL)
FOR INTRAMUSCULAR,
SUBCUTANEOUS OR
INTRAVENOUS USE

esi   **ELKINS-SINN, INC. Cherry Hill, NJ 08034**
A subsidiary of A. H. Robins Company

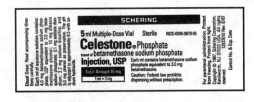

NDC 0173-0350-58
Glaxo
Trandate®
(labetalol hydrochloride)
Injection
5 mg/ml
(100 mg in 20 ml)
For IV injection only.
20 ml Multi-dose Vial   Sterile

Caution: Federal law prohibits dispensing without prescription.
See package insert for Dosage and Administration.
Store between 2° and 30°C (36° and 86°F). Do not freeze.
Protect from light.
Each 1 ml of aqueous solution contains labetalol hydrochloride
5 mg; anhydrous dextrose 45 mg; edetate disodium 0.1 mg;
citric acid monohydrate and sodium hydroxide as necessary to
bring the pH into range; methylparaben 0.8 mg and
propylparaben 0.1 mg as preservatives.
Glaxo Inc.,
Research Triangle Park, NC 27709
Manufactured in England
2/88
4004825

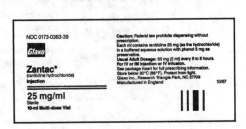

NDC 0173-0363-39
Glaxo
Zantac®
(ranitidine hydrochloride)
Injection
25 mg/ml
Sterile
10-ml Multi-dose Vial

Caution: Federal law prohibits dispensing without
prescription.
Each ml contains ranitidine 25 mg (as the hydrochloride)
in a buffered aqueous solution with phenol 5 mg as
preservative.
Usual Adult Dosage: 50 mg (2 ml) every 6 to 8 hours.
For IV or IM injection or IV infusion.
See package insert for full prescribing information.
Store below 30°C (86°F). Protect from light.
Glaxo Inc., Research Triangle Park, NC 27709
Manufactured in England   10/87

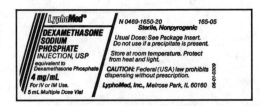

SCHERING
5 ml Multiple-Dose Vial   Sterile   NDC-0085-0679-05
Celestone® Phosphate
brand of betamethasone sodium phosphate
Injection, USP
Total Amount 15 mg
1 ml = 3 mg
Each ml contains betamethasone sodium
phosphate equivalent to 3.0 mg
betamethasone.
Caution: Federal law prohibits
dispensing without prescription.

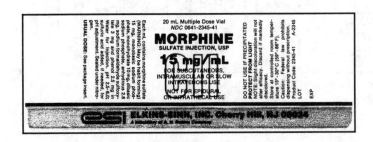

20 mL Multiple Dose Vial
NDC 0641-2345-41
MORPHINE
SULFATE INJECTION, USP
15 mg/mL
FOR SUBCUTANEOUS,
INTRAMUSCULAR OR SLOW
INTRAVENOUS USE
NOT FOR EPIDURAL
OR INTRATHECAL USE

esi   ELKINS-SINN, INC. Cherry Hill, NJ 08034

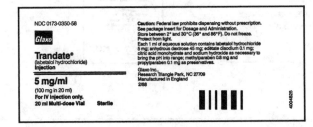

LyphoMed®
**DEXAMETHASONE
SODIUM
PHOSPHATE**
INJECTION, USP
equivalent to
Dexamethasone Phosphate
4 mg/mL
For IV or IM Use.
5 mL Multiple Dose Vial

N 0469-1650-20   165-05
Sterile, Nonpyrogenic
Usual Dose: See Package Insert.
Do not use if a precipitate is present.
Store at room temperature. Protect
from heat and light.
CAUTION: Federal (USA) law prohibits
dispensing without prescription.
LyphoMed, Inc., Melrose Park, IL 60160

PART III

32. Prepare a 4 mg dosage of Trilafon® _____

33. A 60 mg dosage of phenytoin is ordered _____

34. A dosage of 70 mg of gentamicin has been ordered _____

35. Prepare a dosage of clindamycin 180 mg _____

36. Prepare a 750 u dosage of heparin measured to hundredths _____

37. Draw up a 60 mEq dosage of potassium chloride for addition to IV solution

_____

38. 400,000 u of penicillin G has been ordered _____

39. Prepare morphine gr ⅛ _____

40. A dosage of sodium bicarbonate 35 mEq has been ordered for addition to an IV

solution _____

ANSWERS

1. 1.3 mL   **2.** 0.75 mL   **3.** 1.5 mL   **4.** 1.6 mL   **5.** 1.4 mL   **6.** 1.2 mL   **7.** 1.2 mL   **8.** 2.4 mL   **9.** 0.7 mL   **10.** 0.8 mL
11. 2 mL   **12.** 12 mL   **13.** 3 mL   **14.** 4 mL   **15.** 2.6 mL   **16.** 4 mL   **17.** 1.4 mL   **18.** 20 mL   **19.** 16 mL   **20.** 0.5 mL
21. 1.5 mL   **22.** 40 mL   **23.** 1.5 mL   **24.** 0.8 mL   **25.** 2.5 mL   **26.** 1.6 mL   **27.** 0.8 cc   **28.** 1.6 mL   **29.** 2.5 mL   **30.** 20 mL
31. 0.67 mL   **32.** 0.8 mL   **33.** 1.2 mL   **34.** 1.8 mL   **35.** 1.2 mL   **36.** 0.75 mL   **37.** 30 mL   **38.** 1.3 mL   **39.** 0.5 cc   **40.** 35 mL

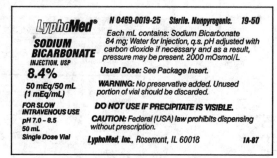

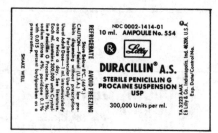

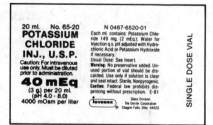

NDC 0009-0268-01
10 ml

**Heparin Sodium
Injection, USP**

Sterile Solution

1,000 Units per ml

from beef lung

For subcutaneous or
intravenous use

Upjohn

See package insert for complete
product information.

Store at controlled room temperature
15°-30° C (59°-86° F)

Each ml contains: heparin sodium,
1,000 USP Units. Also, sodium
chloride, 9 mg; benzyl alcohol,
9.45 mg added as preservative.

811 317 201

The Upjohn Company
Kalamazoo, MI 49001, USA

N 0467-5152-01

20 ml. No. 515-20

**GENTAMICIN
SULFATE
INJ., U.S.P.**

40 mg. per ml.

(pH 3.0 - 5.5)

Invenex

FOR I.V. OR I.M. USE

Each ml contains: Gentamicin Sulfate, U.S.P.
equivalent to 40 mg gentamicin base. Methyl-
paraben 1.8 mg . Propylparaben 0.2 mg . Sodium
Bisulfite 3.2 mg . Edetate Disodium 0.1 mg ;
Water for Injection q.s. pH adjusted with Sodium
Hydroxide or Sulfuric Acid if neccessary.
Usual Dose: See Insert.
Warning: Use only if solution is clear and seal
intact. Sterile.
Caution: Federal law prohibits dispensing without
prescription.   E-82

Gibco Division
The Dexter Corporation
© Chagrin Falls, Ohio 44022

MULTIPLE DOSE VIAL

LyphoMed®

**PHENYTOIN
SODIUM
INJECTION, USP**
100 mg (50 mg/mL)
**FOR IV (No Infusion)
or IM USE**
SINGLE DOSE
Discard Unused Portion
Store at 15°-30°C (59°-86°F)
N 0469-0615-25
2 mL   No. 615-82
LyphoMed, Inc.
Rosemont, IL 60018   K-68

---

5 mg / 1 ml

Trilafon®

brand of
perphenazine
injection, USP

Schering Corporation
Kenilworth, NJ 07033

Control No. & Exp. Date

NDC 0009-0728-05
6505-01-246-8718

60 ml Pharmacy
Bulk Package

Not for direct infusion

Cleocin Phosphate®
Sterile Solution
clindamycin phosphate injection, USP
Equivalent to clindamycin

150 mg per ml

For intramuscular or intravenous use

Caution: Federal law prohibits
dispensing without prescription.

Upjohn   The Upjohn Company
Kalamazoo, MI 49001, USA

15
Measuring Insulin Dosages

OBJECTIVES
The student will
1. distinguish between insulins of animal and human origin
2. discuss the difference between rapid, intermediate and long acting insulins
3. read insulin labels to identify origin and type
4. read calibrations on U-100 insulin syringes
5. measure single insulin dosages
6. measure combined insulin dosages

INTRODUCTION
Insulin dosages are measured in units (u), with the 100 u per cc (U-100) strength being used almost exclusively. Dosages are measured using **special insulin syringes which are calibrated to match the dosage strength of insulin being used**. For example U-100 syringes are used to prepare U-100 strength dosages. This chapter will show you a variety of U-100 syringes to illustrate how to measure dosages. However, let's begin with an introduction to the types of insulin in use.

• TYPES OF INSULIN •

Insulins are classified by origin (animal or human) and by action (rapid, intermediate or long acting). The origin or source of insulins is printed on every label, and it is important to know where to locate this information as many physicians specify origin when writing insulin orders. Refer to figures 55 and 56. Notice the small print on the Regular insulin label in figure 55 which identifies its pork (animal) origin, and the Regular insulin label in figure 56 which identifies its human (semi-synthetic) origin. Also notice how similiar these labels are. Careful reading of labels is essential for correct identification.

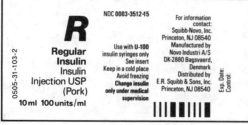

Figure 55

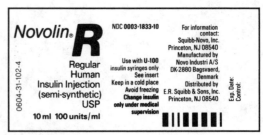

Figure 56

Next look at the labels in figures 57 and 58. Both of these insulins are of human origin and use the trade name Humulin®. Notice the initials which follow the trade name: L and U. These identify the type of insulin by action time. There are three basic action times of insulins. Regular and Semilente have the most rapid action, beginning in ½ hr, peaking in 2½–5 hr, and ending in 8 hr. In the intermediate range are the Lente and NPH insulins, beginning in 1½–2½ hr, peaking in 4–15 hr, and ending in 16–24 hr. Among the long acting insulins are the Ultralente and Protamine Zinc, beginning in 4 hr, peaking in 10–30 hr, and ending in 36 hr. Insulin types and dosages are prescribed to correlate with life style, diet and activity schedule.

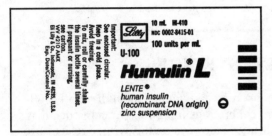

Figure 57   Figure 58

PROBLEM

Identify the type and origin of the insulin whose labels are reproduced below.

Type of Insulin	Origin
1. _____	_____
2. _____	_____
3. _____	_____
4. _____	_____
5. _____	_____
6. _____	_____

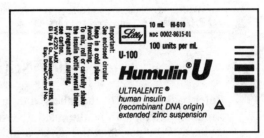

5

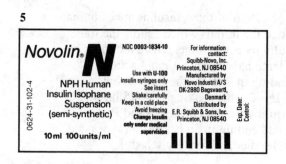

6

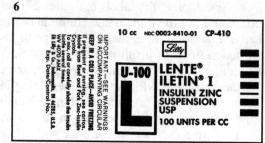

ANSWERS   **1.** Ultralente; beef   **2.** NPH; beef and pork   **3.** Buffered Regular; human   **4.** Semilente; beef
5. NPH; human   **6.** Lente; beef and pork

• U-100 INSULIN SYRINGES •

Refer back to each of the labels you have just read and notice that all have a U-100 strength. Then examine the insulin syringe calibrations in figure 59, and notice that this is a 100 u per cc scale. The warning printed sideways on the syringe reads "use U-100 insulin only." **For U-100 insulin dosage measurement you must use a U-100 calibrated syringe.**

There are several sizes (capacities) of U-100 syringes in use. The easiest of these to read and use are the Lo-Dose® syringes, which have a capacity of 30 or 50 u. Refer to the calibrations in figure 60 for a 50 u Lo-Dose syringe. Lo-Dose syringes do exactly what their name implies: they measure low dosages, but on an enlarged and easier to read scale. This larger scale is an important safety feature for diabetic patients, who frequently have vision problems, and for ease of use by medical personnel.

Refer again to the calibrations of the 50 u (½ cc) capacity syringe in figure 60. Notice that each calibration measures 1 u with each 5 u increment being numbered.

Figure 59

PROBLEM

Refer to the syringe calibrations for 50 u Lo-Dose syringes below and identify the dosages indicated by the arrows.

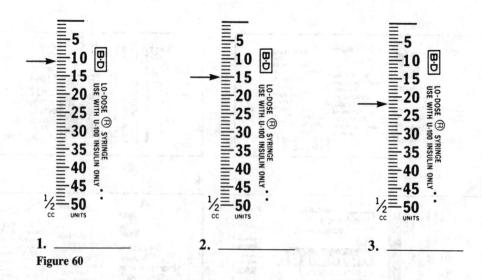

1. _____   2. _____   3. _____

Figure 60

ANSWERS   **1.** 11 u   **2.** 15 u   **3.** 22 u

PROBLEM

Use the U-100 Lo-Dose calibrations in figure 61 to measure the following dosages. Have your instructor check your accuracy.

1. 33 u   **2.** 38 u   **3.** 18 u

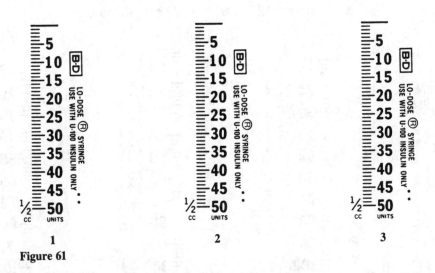

Figure 61

There are two 1 cc (100 u) capacity syringes in common use. Refer to the first of these in figure 62. Notice the 100 u (1 cc) capacity, and that each 10 u increment is numbered, 10, 20 etc. Next notice the number of calibrations in each 10 u increment, which is five, indicating that **this syringe is calibrated in 2 u increments. Odd numbered units are measured between the even calibrations.** For example the arrow on syringe 4 identifies 85 u.

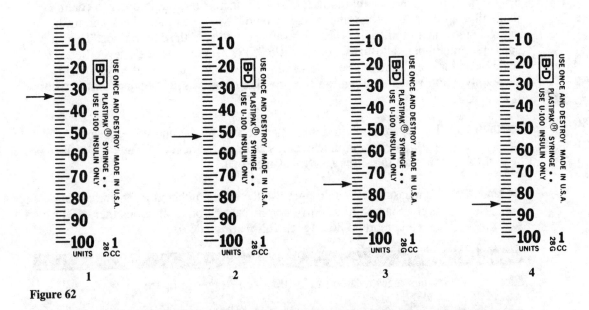

Figure 62

PROBLEM

Identify the dosages on the following U-100 1 cc syringes in figure 62.

1. _____   **2.** _____   **3.** _____

ANSWERS   **1.** 33 u   **2.** 52 u   **3.** 75 u

PROBLEM

Draw an arrow on the syringes in figure 63 to measure the following dosages.

1. 67 u   **2.** 84 u   **3.** 28 u   **4.** 45 u

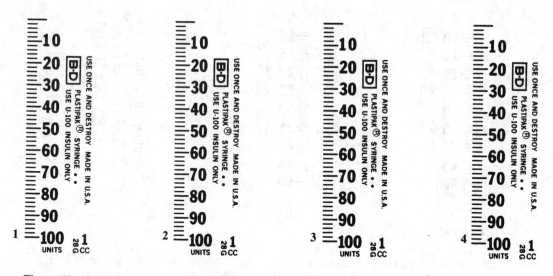

Figure 63

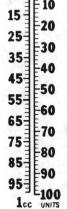

Figure 64

The second type of U-100 1 cc capacity syringe is illustrated in figure 64. Notice that this syringe has a double scale, the odd numbers are on the left, and the even are on the right. Each 5 u increment is numbered, but on opposite sides of the syringe. This syringe does have a calibration for each 1 u increment, but in order to count them all to measure a dosage, the syringe would have to be rotated back and forth, which could cause confusion. There is a safer way to read the calibrations. To measure uneven numbered dosages, for example 7, 13, 27, etc., use the uneven (left) scale only; for even numbered dosages such as 6, 10, 56, etc., use the even (right) scale only. **Count each calibration (on one side only) as 2 u, because that is what it is measuring.**

EXAMPLE 1   To prepare an 89 u dosage start at 85 u on the uneven left scale, count the first calibration above this as 87 u, the next as 89 u (**each calibration on the same side measures 2 u**).

EXAMPLE 2   To measure a 26 u dosage, use the even numbered right side calibrations. Start at 20 u, move up one calibration to 22 u, another to 24 u, and one more to 26 u (**each calibration is 2 u**).

PROBLEM

Identify the dosages measured on the U-100 1 cc syringes in figure 65.

1. _____   **2.** _____   **3.** _____

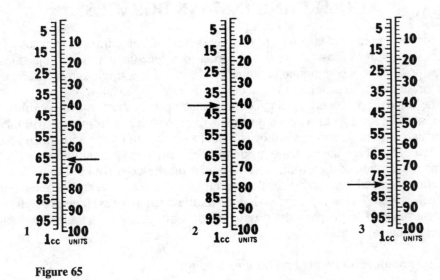

Figure 65

ANSWERS   **1.** 66 u   **2.** 41 u   **3.** 79 u

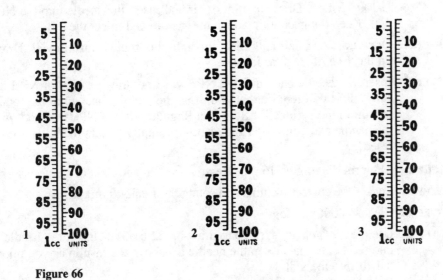

Figure 66

PROBLEM

Draw an arrow on each U-100 syringe in figure 66 to identify the following dosages.

1. 55 u   **2.** 94 u   **3.** 69 u

• COMBINING INSULIN DOSAGES •

Insulin dependent individuals must have at least one and sometimes several sub-cutaneous injections of insulin per day. In order to reduce the number of injections as much as possible it is common to combine two insulins in a single syringe, for example a short acting with either an intermediate or long acting insulin.

The standard procedure used to combine insulins is to **draw up the regular insulin into the syringe first**. Both insulins will be withdrawn from sealed 10 mL vials, which require that an amount of air equal to the insulin to be withdrawn be injected first. This keeps the pressure inside the vial equalized. An additional step concerns preparation of the insulin itself. Regular insulin does not need to be mixed, but intermediate and long acting insulins precipitate out. They need to be rotated and mixed before withdrawal from the vial. **The smallest capacity syringe possible should be selected to prepare the dosage**, as the enlarged scale is easier and therefore more accurate to read.

The procedure for combining insulins is as follows:

EXAMPLE 1   A dosage of 10 u of Regular and 48 u of NPH insulin has been ordered.

STEP 1. Locate the correct insulins and rotate the NPH until it is thoroughly mixed.

STEP 2. Use an alcohol wipe to cleanse both vial tops.

STEP 3. The combined dosage (10 u + 48 u = 58 u) requires the use of a 1 cc U-100 syringe. Draw up 48 u of air and insert the needle into the NPH vial. Keep the needle tip above the insulin and inject the air.

STEP 4. Draw up 10 u of air and inject this into the Regular insulin vial. Draw up the 10 u of Regular insulin.

STEP 5. Insert the needle back into the NPH vial and draw up 48 u of NPH insulin. This will require that you draw the plunger back until the total insulin in the syringe is 58 u (10 u Regular + 48 u NPH). Withdraw the needle and administer the insulin promptly so that the NPH does not resettle.

EXAMPLE 2   The order is to give 16 u of Regular insulin and 22 u of Lente insulin.

STEP 1. Locate the correct insulins and rotate the Lente to mix it.

STEP 2. Cleanse both vial tops

STEP 3. Use a 50 u capacity syringe to draw up 22 u of air. Insert the needle into the Lente vial. Keep the needle tip above the insulin as you inject the air into the vial.

STEP 4. Draw up 16 u of air and inject it into the Regular insulin vial. Draw up the 16 u of Regular insulin.

STEP 5. Insert the needle back into the Lente vial and draw up Lente insulin until the syringe capacity is 38 u (16 U Regular + 22 u Lente). Administer the dosage promptly.

PROBLEM

For each of the following combined insulin dosages indicate the total volume of the combined dosage, and the smallest capacity syringe you can use to prepare it (30 u, 50 u and 100 u capacity syringes are available).

	Total Volume	Syringe Size
1. 28 u Regular, 64 u NPH	_____	_____
2. 16 u Ultralente, 6 u Regular	_____	_____
3. 33 u Regular, 41 u Lente	_____	_____
4. 21 u Regular, 52 u NPH	_____	_____
5. 13 u Regular, 27 u Ultralente	_____	_____

ANSWERS **1.** 92 u; 100 u   **2.** 22 u; 30 u   **3.** 74 u; 100 u   **4.** 73 u; 100 u   **5.** 40 u; 50 u

A U-40 strength of insulin is also still being manufactured, but is used on a more limited basis. If you encounter this strength of insulin it is necessary to obtain U-40 calibrated syringes to measure dosages.

This concludes the chapter on measuring insulin dosages. The important points to remember from this chapter are:

- insulin vial labels must be read carefully to identify type and origin of the insulin

- the U-100 insulins are measured using U-100 calibrated syringes

- the smallest capacity syringe possible is used for ease and accuracy of dosage preparation

- dosages on U-100 1 cc capacity syringes are measured in 2 u increments, while on 30 u and 50 u syringes they are measured in 1 u increments

- when insulin dosages are combined the Regular insulin is drawn up first

- the intermediate and long acting insulins precipitate out and must be thoroughly mixed before measurement

SUMMARY SELF TEST

Measuring Insulin Dosages

DIRECTIONS Use the syringe calibrations provided to measure the following dosages. For combined insulin dosages indicate the exact calibration to be used for each insulin ordered.

1. 37 u Regular

2. 17 u Regular
   12 u Lente

3. 48 u NPH

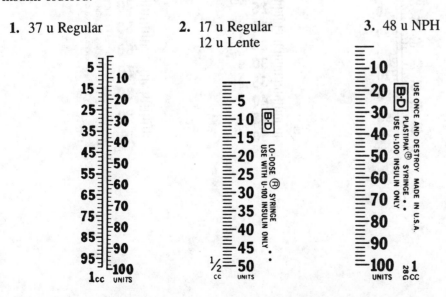

4. 14 u Regular
58 u NPH

5. 12 u NPH

6. 18 u Regular
8 u Lente

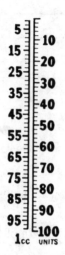

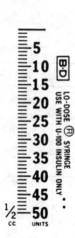

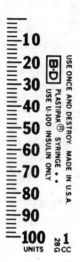

7. 23 u Regular
14 u Humulin BR

8. 8 u Regular
20 u Protamine Zinc

9. 23 u Lente

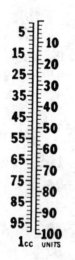

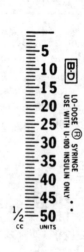

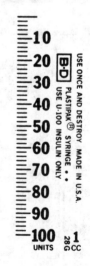

10. 57 u NPH

11. 22 u Regular
8 u Lente

12. 15 u Regular
43 u NPH

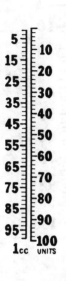

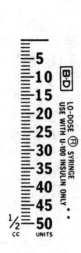

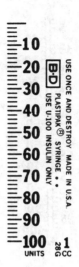

13. 24 u Regular
27 u Semilente

14. 33 u Regular
10 u Humulin L

15. 55 u Regular

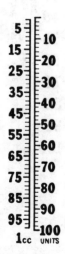

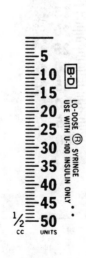

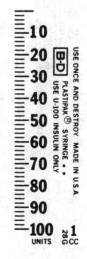

DIRECTIONS   Identify the dosages measured on the following syringes.

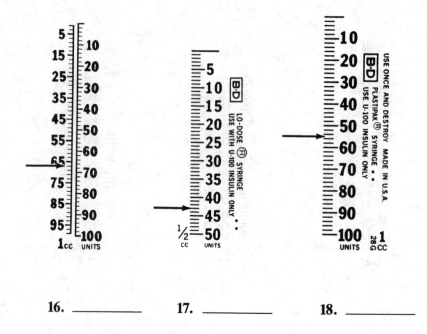

16. _____   17. _____   18. _____

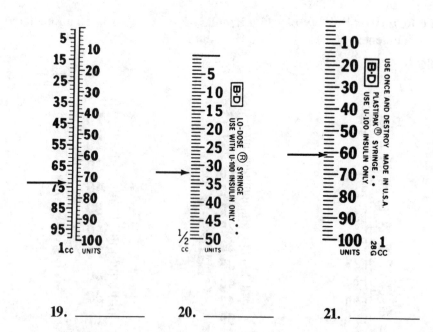

19. _____   20. _____   21. _____

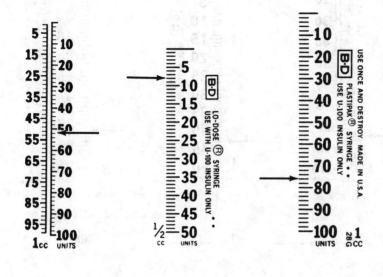

22. _____   23. _____   24. _____

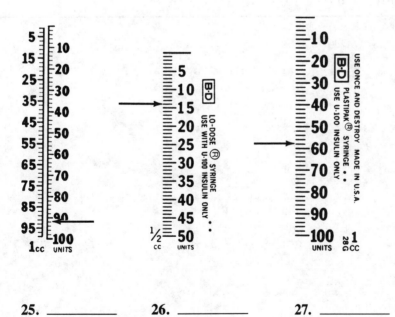

25. _____   26. _____   27. _____

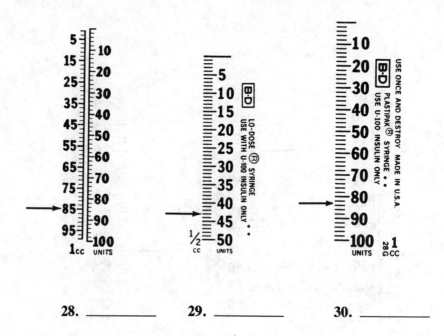

28. _____   29. _____   30. _____

SECTION
FIVE

Medication Administration Systems

Veterans Administration — CONTINUING MEDICATION RECORD

MONTH: MAY   YEAR: 19__

ORIG. ORD. DATE	START DATE	STOP DATE	MEDICATIONS DOSE/ROUTE/FREQUENCY	ADMIN. TIMES:	3	4	5	6	7	8	9	10	11	12	13	14	15	16
5-1	5-1	5-15	Furosemide 40mg P.o. b.i.d.	0900 MC / 1700														
5-1	5-1	5-15	Ferrous sulfate 300mg p.o. q.d.	0900 MC														
5-1	5-1	5-20	Allopurinal 300mg p.o. b.i.d.	0900 MC / 1700														
5-3	5-3	5-18	Digoxin 0.25mg p.o. q.d.	0900 MC / 64 MP														
5-3	5-3	5-13	Gentamicin 40mg IM t.i.l.	0900 MC / 1300 / 2100														

SIGNATURE/TITLE: Maria Clark Rn

INIT.	ALLERGIES
MC	

ADDRESSOGRAPH

PATIENT Identification

INJECTION SITES

INDICATE RIGHT (R) OR LEFT (L)
1. DELTOID
2. ABDOMEN
3. ILIAC CREST
4. GLUTEAL
5. THIGH

VA FORM 10-2970
AUG 1982

SUPERSEDES VA FORM 10-2970, JAN 1973, WHICH WILL NOT BE USED.

NAME: BED #   PAGE____OF____

16

Medication Administration Records

OBJECTIVES

The student will read medication records to identify
1. drugs ordered on a continuing basis
2. dosage ordered
3. time of administration
4. route of administration

INTRODUCTION

The most widely used system of drug administration currently used in hospitals is the medication record system. In this system all the drugs a patient is receiving on a continuing basis are listed on a single record. In some hospitals p.r.n. and IV medications are also listed on this record, in others these are on a separate record, or records. A wide variety of records are in use, and the purpose of this chapter is to provide an introduction to a sufficient number so that you will not be confused by the differences, but rather will recognize and locate essential information which is common to all. The focus will be on identifying the drug, dosage, time and route of medications being administered on a continuing basis.

• MEDICATION RECORD 1 •

On the opposite page is the Continuing Medication Record currently being used at Veterans Hospitals in the U.S.A. Notice that from left to right the columns identify the original order date of the drug; the date administration was started; the date the order expires; the drug name, dosage, route and frequency of administration; the time of administration; and finally, the date columns used by the person administering to initial, indicating that the dosage was given. For example, Maria Clark has initialed for the 0900 dosages on May 3rd, and has identified her initials in the Signature/Title column on the lower right of the form. This hospital uses the 24 hour military time clock (0–2400).

Refer back to the drug information. The first drug, furosemide 40 mg, has been ordered p.o. b.i.d., to be given at 0900 and 1700. The administration time column is set up beginning with the earliest administration for the day, and includes all dosages to be given on a continuing basis. The patient identification would be stamped in the lower left corner.

PROBLEM

Read the VA record and identify for each drug listed the name, dosage, route and time of administration.

TORONTO GENERAL HOSPITAL   **MEDICATION ADMINISTRATION RECORD**   PAGE ___1___ OF ___1___

Instructions
1. Fill in allergies, diagnosis, and number of pages being used at one time if applicable.
2. Sign and initial legend below.
3. Initial off meds as they are administered.
4. For more detailed information refer to TGH Nursing Procedures.
5. Retain completed original in chart.

NURSE NAME (PLEASE PRINT)	INITIALS	NURSE NAME (PLEASE PRINT)	INITIALS	NURSE NAME (PLEASE PRINT)	INITIALS
M. Bennie	MB				
				M. Williams	M.W.
				WARD SECRETARY	

PATIENT IDENTIFICATION

ALLERGIES
NONE KNOWN ☒

SCHEDULED MEDICATIONS

DIAGNOSIS	TIME	DATE 15	DATE 16	DATE 17	DATE 18	DATE 19
O.A. TOTAL HIP REPLACEMENT						
TRANSCRIBED/RECOPIED BY M.W. — DRUG Digoxin — DOSE 0.125 mg	0900	MB Apical R.				
CHECKED BY (RN) MB — FREQUENCY & ADDITIONAL DIRECTIONS 9 a.m. — ROUTE PO		72				
CHECKED BY (PHM) LQ — DATE ORDERED Oct 14 — AUTO STOP DATE — COMMENTS						
TRANSCRIBED/RECOPIED BY M.W. — DRUG DoCusate Sodium cap ī — DOSE	0900	MB				
CHECKED BY (RN) MB — FREQUENCY & ADDITIONAL DIRECTIONS b.i.d. — ROUTE PO	1800					
CHECKED BY (PHM) LQ — DATE ORDERED Oct 14 — AUTO STOP DATE — COMMENTS						
TRANSCRIBED/RECOPIED BY M.W. — DRUG Ancef — DOSE 1 g	0600					
CHECKED BY (RN) MB — FREQUENCY & ADDITIONAL DIRECTIONS q.i.d. — ROUTE IV	1200 / 1800	MB				
CHECKED BY (PHM) LQ — DATE ORDERED Oct 14 — AUTO STOP DATE — COMMENTS	2400					
TRANSCRIBED/RECOPIED BY M.W. — DRUG FERSAMEL — DOSE 200 mg	0900	MB				
CHECKED BY (RN) MB — FREQUENCY & ADDITIONAL DIRECTIONS t.i.D. — ROUTE P.O.	1400	MB				
CHECKED BY (PHM) LQ — DATE ORDERED Oct 14 — AUTO STOP DATE — COMMENTS	1800					
TRANSCRIBED/RECOPIED BY — DRUG — DOSE						
CHECKED BY (RN) — FREQUENCY & ADDITIONAL DIRECTIONS — ROUTE						
CHECKED BY (PHM) — DATE ORDERED — AUTO STOP DATE — COMMENTS						
TRANSCRIBED/RECOPIED BY — DRUG — DOSE						
CHECKED BY (RN) — FREQUENCY & ADDITIONAL DIRECTIONS — ROUTE						
CHECKED BY (PHM) — DATE ORDERED — AUTO STOP DATE — COMMENTS						
TRANSCRIBED/RECOPIED BY — DRUG — DOSE						
CHECKED BY (RN) — FREQUENCY & ADDITIONAL DIRECTIONS — ROUTE						
CHECKED BY (PHM) — DATE ORDERED — AUTO STOP DATE — COMMENTS						

PLEASE PRESS FIRMLY WITH BALL POINT PEN   **CHART ORIGINAL**   TGH 610 (12/84)

	DRUG	DOSAGE	ROUTE	TIME
1.	_____	_____	_____	_____
2.	_____	_____	_____	_____
3.	_____	_____	_____	_____
4.	_____	_____	_____	_____
5.	_____	_____	_____	_____

6. If it was your responsibility to administer the drugs to this patient at 1700, which ones would you give?_____

ANSWERS **1.** furosemide 40 mg p.o. 0900, 1700 **2.** ferrous sulfate 300 mg p.o. 0900 **3.** allopurinal 300 mg p.o. 0900, 1700 **4.** digoxin 0.25 mg p.o. 0900 **5.** gentamicin 40 mg IM 0900, 1300, 2100 **6.** At 1700 you would give furosemide 40 mg p.o., and allopurinal 300 mg p.o.

• MEDICATION RECORD 2 •

Take a close look at the record on the opposite page from the Toronto General Hospital. You can see that the information it contains is very similar to the VA record, only the arrangement is different. Patient identification is at the upper right, nurse signature identification upper left. The continuing medications are listed on the left, with the time and date of administration columns to the right. This medical center also uses military time.

PROBLEM

Read the TGH record and list the drug, dosage, route, and time of the drugs given by MB (M. Bennie) on October 15th.

ANSWERS digoxin 0.125 mg p.o. 0900; docusate sodium caps 1 p.o. 0900; Ancef 1 g IV 1200; Fersamel 200 mg p.o. 0900 and 1400

MEDICATION ADMINISTRATION RECORD

PATIENT IDENTIFICATION

DIAGNOSES: _____

ALLERGIC TO: _____   DIET: _____
(Record in Red)

Scheduled Medications

OR. DATE / INITIALS	EXP.DATE / TIME	MEDICATION-DOSAGE-FREQUENCY-RT. OF ADM.	HR.	5/2	5/3	5/4	5/5	5/6	5/7	5/8	5/9	5/10
5-2 MC	5-16 p̄ 12N	TAGAMET 300 mg (p.o.) q6°	6									
			12									
			6									
			12									
5-2 MC	5-16 p̄ 9A	BLOCADREN 10 mg (p.o.) b.id.	9									
			9									
5-2 MC	5-16 p̄ 6P	NITRO-BID UNG 1" (TOP) APPLY TO CHEST q.6° WHILE AWAKE	6									
			12									
			6									
			12									
5-2 MC	5-16 p̄ 6P	DIALOSE CAP ī (p.o.) t.i.d.	9									
			1									
			9									
5-2 MC	5-16 p̄ 6A	BACTRIM DS ī (p.o.) b.id.	6									
			6									

DATES GIVEN

USE RED ASTERISK *TO INDICATE DOSES
NOT GIVEN - EXPLAIN IN NURSE'S NOTES

Single Orders + Pre-Operatives

OR. DATE / INITIALS	MEDICATION-DOSAGE-RT. OF ADM.	TO BE GIVEN DATE	TIME	NURSE INITIAL	OR. DATE INITIALS	MEDICATION-DOSAGE-RT. OF ADM.

AGE _____ RELIGION _____ DOCTOR _____ DATE/TIME ADMITTED _____

RM. _____ NAME _____

Lionville Systems, Inc.
© Parke, Davis & Company, 1978
P/N 10104 Rev. H

• MEDICATION RECORD 3 •

Medication record 3 is produced by Lionville Systems of Parke-Davis & Co. Notice that it provides space at the lower left for Single Order and Pre-Operative drugs. The previous records you examined listed these, and p.r.n. drugs, on separate records. IV drugs are also often listed on separate records. The nurse signature identification is not shown, as it is on the back of this particular form.

PROBLEM

Read the medication record on the opposite page and list the drug, dosage, and route of each drug that will be administered at 6 p.m.

ANSWERS   Tagamet 300 mg p.o.; Nitro-Bid ung 1″ topical to chest; Bactrim DS 1 p.o.

ROUTINE MEDICATION ORDERS

Start / Stop	Medication and Dose	Schedule	Route / Nurse		Date 5-3	Date 5-4	Date 5-5	Date 5-6
5-1	RESPBID 300mg t.i.d.	08 14 20	p.o. MC.	Time Site Initials				
				Time Site Initials				
				Time Site Initials				
				Time Site Initials				
				Time Site Initials				
				Time Site Initials				
				Time Site Initials				

Initials	Signature	Initials	Signature
MC	M. Clark RN.		

UNIVERSITY HOSPITAL
UNIVERSITY OF CALIFORNIA MEDICAL CENTER
SAN DIEGO

MEDICATION ADMINISTRATION RECORD

Physician

Allergies

Room #   Name

• MEDICATION RECORD 4 •

The final record, from the University of California Medical Center, San Diego, also uses military time. Once again you can see the similarities with the previous records reproduced. Examine this record before completing the following problem.

PROBLEM

Use the drug entry on Medication Record 4 as reference to enter the following drugs, dosages, frequency, and route of administration on the form. Record you initials in the ''Nurse'' column to indicate you have done the transcribing, and identify your initials appropriately on the record. Have your instructor check your accuracy.

1. Lanoxin 0.25 mg p.o. q.d. 0900
2. Lasix 20 mg p.o. q.a.m. 0900
3. Slow-K 2 tabs p.o. b.i.d. 0900, 1800
4. Claforan 1 g IV q.6.h. 0600, 1200, 1800, 2400
5. Medihaler-Iso 1–2 inhalations q.i.d. 0800, 1400, 1800, 2200

This concludes the chapter on Medication Administration Records. The important points to remember from this chapter are:

- all the drugs the patient is receiving on a continuing basis are entered on this record

- the record contains a column for each date, and a time block to record each dosage ordered

- the person administering the medications is responsible for entering her/his initials in the appropriate time block for each dosage, and for identifying her/his initials on the record

17
Medication Card Administration

OBJECTIVES
The student will read medication cards to identify
1. drug
2. dosage
3. time of administration
4. route of administration

INTRODUCTION
In the medication card system a separate card is made for each drug the patient is to receive. These are usually combined with the medicine cards for all other patients on a unit, and stored in a card rack under the time of next administration. If your assignment was to give the 9 a.m. medications you would pull all the cards from the 9 a.m. slot, prepare, administer, and chart them, then sort and return the cards once again to the time slot of the next administration; 1 p.m., 9 p.m., and so on.

There are several recognized weaknesses in this system, lost or misplaced cards being one of the more serious. For this reason many hospitals are phasing the system out in favor of the medication record system. However, you will still need to know how to read a medicine card correctly.

• READING MEDICATION CARDS •

Examine the medication cards labeled A and B in figure 67. Notice that both cards contain the patient's name, surname first. The room and bed number (frequently written in pencil, so that it can be changed if the patient is moved) is next. Both contain the name of the drug, acetaminophen, the dosage, 600 mg, and the frequency and route of administration, t.i.d. p.o. The time of administration is designated by an X in the appropriate time slot. The shaded areas on these cards identify the evening/night hours. Card B has a built-in weakness in that the time of administration is X'ed in a separate column, leaving open the possibility of misreading the 2100 dosage, for example, as 0900 (this card uses military time).

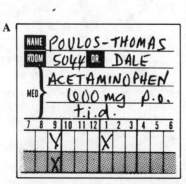
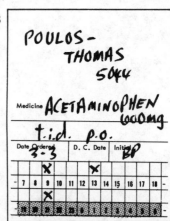

Figure 67

This information is all you will need to read medication cards. The important points to remember from this chapter are:

- in the medication card system a card is made for each drug the patient is to receive

- the patient's name, room number, drug, dosage, frequency and route of administration are all printed on the card

- the time of administration is X'ed in the appropriate time space for each dosage to be administered

SUMMARY SELF TEST
Medication Card Administration

DIRECTIONS For each of the following medication cards identify the drug, dosage, route and time of administration. Indicate a.m. or p.m. for dosages given at standard time, but omit these designations if military time is used.

	DRUG	DOSAGE	ROUTE	TIME
1.				
2.				
3.				
4.				
5.				
6.				
7.				
8.				
9.				
10.				
11.				
12.				

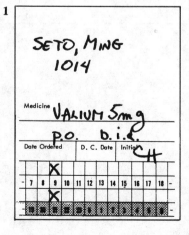

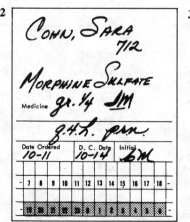

3

YOUNG, DENNIS
43 A

Medicine COMPAZINE 10mg
q4h PRN IM

Date Ordered	D. C. Date	Initial

4

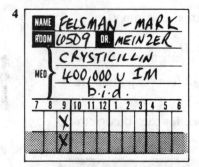

NAME FELSMAN - MARK
ROOM 0509 DR. MEINZER
MED CRYSTICILLIN
400,000 u IM
b·i·d.

7 8 9 10 11 12 1 2 3 4 5 6

5

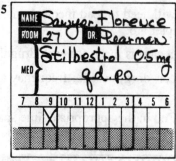

NAME Sawyer, Florence
ROOM 27 DR. Pearman
MED Stilbestrol 0.5mg
qd. po.

7 8 9 10 11 12 1 2 3 4 5 6

6

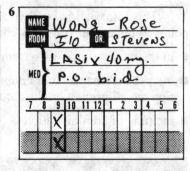

NAME WONG - ROSE
ROOM 510 DR. STEVENS
MED LASix 40mg.
P.O. b·i·d.

7 8 9 10 11 12 1 2 3 4 5 6

7

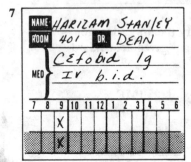

NAME HARIZAM STANLEY
ROOM 401 DR. DEAN
MED Cefobid 1g
IV b·i·d.

7 8 9 10 11 12 1 2 3 4 5 6

8

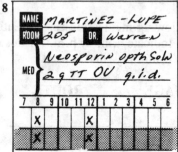

NAME MARTINEZ - LUPE
ROOM 205 DR. Warren
MED Neosporin opth Soln
2 g TT OU q·i·d.

7 8 9 10 11 12 1 2 3 4 5 6

9

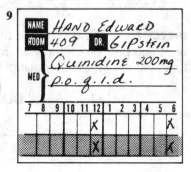

NAME HAND Edward
ROOM 409 DR. GIPstein
MED Quinidine 200mg
p.o. q·i·d.

7 8 9 10 11 12 1 2 3 4 5 6

10

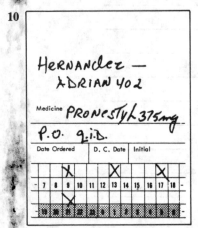

HERNANdez —
ADRIAN 402

Medicine PRONESTYL 375mg
P.O. q·i·d.

Date Ordered	D. C. Date	Initial

- 7 8 9 10 11 12 13 14 15 16 17 18

11

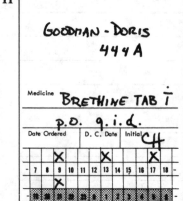

GOODMAN - DORIS
444 A

Medicine BRETHINE TAB Ī
p.o. q·i·d.

Date Ordered	D. C. Date	Initial

- 7 8 9 10 11 12 13 14 15 16 17 18

12

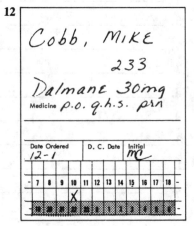

Cobb, MIKE
233
Dalmane 30mg
Medicine p.o. q.h.s. prn

Date Ordered	D. C. Date	Initial
12-1		mc

- 7 8 9 10 11 12 13 14 15 16 17 18

ANSWERS

1.	Valium	5 mg	po	0900-2100
2.	morphine sulfate	gr ¼	IM	q.4.h. p.r.n.
3.	Compazine	10 mg	IM	q.4.h. p.r.n.
4.	Crysticillin	400,000 u	IM	9-9
5.	stilbestrol	0.5 mg	p.o.	9 a.m.
6.	Lasix	40 mg	p.o.	9-9
7.	Cefobid	1 g	IV	9-9
8.	Neosporin opth. soln.	2 gtt	OU	8-12-8-12
9.	quinidine	200 mg	p.o.	6-12-6-12
10.	Pronestyl	375 mg	p.o.	0900-1300-1700-2100
11.	Brethine	1 tab	p.o.	0900-1300-1700-2100
12.	Dalmane	30 mg	p.o.	2200 p.r.n.

SECTION

SIX

Pediatric Medications

18
Pediatric Dosage Calculation by Body Weight: mg per kg

OBJECTIVES
The student will
1. convert body weight from lb to kg
2. convert body weight from kg to lb
3. calculate dosages using mg/kg, mg/lb
4. determine if dosages ordered are within normal range for each child

INTRODUCTION
The most common way in which pediatric medications are prescribed is on the basis of a child's body weight. Dosages are expressed in terms of mg/kg/day, or mg/lb/day. The total daily dosage is usually administered in divided (more than one) doses per day, for example q.6.h., t.i.d., and so on.

The doctor will, of course, order the drug and dosage. However it is a nursing responsibility to check each dosage to be sure the order is correct. Each drug label or drug package insert provides specific dosage details, but more complete information is readily available in drug formularies, the PDR, and other nursing or medical references. The hospital pharmacist is an excellent resource person who can also supply you with additional information.

In this chapter you will learn how to calculate drug dosages based on body weight. However, a preliminary step is necessary to understand conversions between kg and lb, since dosages may be ordered in one, and body weight recorded in the other.

• CONVERSION OF BODY WEIGHT: LB TO KG; KG TO LB •

Many hospitals still record body weight in lb, but most drug literature states dosages in terms of kg. The most common conversion is therefore from lb to kg. **One kg equals 2.2 lb; to convert from lb to kg divide by 2.2.** Since you are dividing, the answer, in kg, will be **smaller** than the lb you are converting. Answers are expressed to the nearest tenth.

EXAMPLE 1   Convert 41 lb to kg

$$41 \text{ lb} = 41 \div 2.2 = \textbf{18.6 kg}$$

Your answer must be a smaller number because you are dividing, and it is (41 lb = 18.6 kg).

EXAMPLE 2   Convert 27 lb to kg

27 lb = 27 ÷ 2.2 = 12.27 = **12.3 kg**

PROBLEM

Convert the following body weights from lb to kg.

    1. 14.5 lb = _____ kg

    2. 19 lb   = _____ kg

    3. 63 lb   = _____ kg

    4. 31 lb   = _____ kg

    5. 59 lb   = _____ kg

ANSWERS   **1.** 6.6 kg   **2.** 8.6 kg   **3.** 28.6 kg   **4.** 14.1 kg   **5.** 26.8 kg

To convert in the opposite direction, from kg to lb, always multiply by 2.2. Because you are multiplying the answer, in lb, will be **larger** than the kg you started with. Express weight to the nearest tenth.

EXAMPLE 1   Convert 23 kg to lb

23 kg = 23 × 2.2 = **50.6 lb**

Your answer must be larger because you are multiplying, and it is, 23 kg = 50.6 lb.

EXAMPLE 2   Convert 14 kg to lb

14 × 2.2 = **30.8 lb**

PROBLEM

Convert the following body weights from kg to lb.

    1. 21 kg = _____ lb

    2. 42 kg = _____ lb

    3. 18 kg = _____ lb

    4. 33 kg = _____ lb

    5. 10 kg = _____ lb

ANSWERS   **1.** 46.2 lb   **2.** 92.4 lb   **3.** 39.6 lb   **4.** 72.6 lb   **5.** 22 lb

• CALCULATING DOSAGES •

Once the child's body weight is expressed in kg or lb to correlate with the dosage specifications, the dosage itself can be calculated. **This is a two step procedure. First calculate the total daily dosage, then divide this by the number of doses to**

be administered. Let's look at an example. Refer to the amoxicillin (Polymox®) label in figure 68.

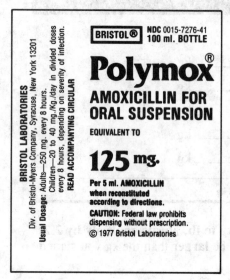

Figure 68

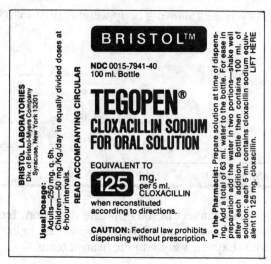

Figure 69

EXAMPLE 1 Refer to the information written sideways on the left of the Polymox® label and obtain the following information.

1. What is the average dosage range in mg/kg/day? _____

2. How is this to be administered? _____

3. Exactly how many doses will be given per day (24 hours)? _____

ANSWERS **1.** 20–40 mg/kg/day   **2.** divided doses every 8 hours   **3.** 24 ÷ 8 hr = 3 doses

Once you have located the dosage information you can move ahead and calculate the dosage. Let's assume you are checking the dosage ordered for an 18 kg child. Start by calculating the safe dosage range.

$$20 \text{ mg} \times 18 \text{ kg} = 360 \text{ mg/day}$$

$$40 \text{ mg} \times 18 \text{ kg} = 720 \text{ mg/day}$$

The safety range for this 18 kg child is **360–720 mg/day**. The drug is to be given in divided doses q.8.h.

$$\text{q.8.h.} = 24 \div 8 = \textbf{3 doses per day}$$

$$360 \text{ mg} \div 3 = 120 \text{ mg per dose}$$

$$720 \text{ mg} \div 3 = 240 \text{ mg per dose}$$

The dosage range is **120 mg to 240 mg per dose q.8.h.** Now that you have the dosage range for this child you are able to assess the accuracy of physician orders. Let's look at some.

1. If the order is to give 125 mg q.8.h. is this a safe dosage? Yes, 125 mg q.8.h. is within the safety range of 120–240 mg per dose.

2. If the order is to give 375 mg q.8.h. is this a safe dosage? No, this is an overdosage. The maximum recommended dosage is 240 mg per dose. The 375 mg dose should not be given; the doctor must be called and the order questioned.

3. If the order is for 75 mg q.8.h. is this a safe dosage? The recommended lower limit for an 18 kg child is 120 mg. While 75 mg might be safe, it will probably be ineffective. Notify the doctor that the dosage appears to be too low.

4. If the order is for 250 mg q.8.h. is this safe? Since 240 mg per dose is the recommended upper safety limit 250 mg q.8.h. is probably safe. The drug strength is 125 mg per 5 mL and a 250 mg dosage is 10 mL. The doctor may have ordered this dosage based on dosage strength and ease of preparation. If you have any doubt call the doctor. **Remember that discrepancies in dosages are much more significant if the number of mg ordered is small.** For example the difference between 4 mg and 6 mg is much more critical than the difference between 240 mg and 250 mg. Additional factors which must be considered are the child's age, weight, and medical condition. While these cannot be dealt with at length keep in mind that the **younger, smaller, or more compromised the child is, the more critical a discrepancy is likely to be**.

5. If the dosage ordered is 125 mg q.4.h. is this a safe dosage? In this order the frequency of administration, q.4.h., does not fit the recommendations of q.8.h. The total daily dosage of 750 mg (125 mg × 6 doses = 750 mg) is higher than the 720 mg maximum. There may be a reason the doctor ordered this dosage but call him to verify the order.

PROBLEM

Refer to the cloxacillin (Tegopen®) label in figure 69 and answer the following questions.

1. What is the average children's dosage? _____

2. How is this dosage to be administered? _____

3. How many divided doses will this be in 24 hours? _____

4. What will the total daily dose be for a child weighing 10 kg? _____

5. The dosage strength of this oral cloxacillin solution is 125 mg per 5 mL, and the doctor has ordered 125 mg q.6.h. for this 10 kg child. Is there any need to question this order? _____

ANSWERS   1. 50 mg/kg/day   **2.** equal doses q.6.h.   **3.** 4 doses in 24 hrs.   **4.** 500 mg   **5.** No

PROBLEM

Refer to the dicloxacillin (Dynapen®) label in figure 70. Answer the following questions regarding dosage for a child weighing 32 kg.

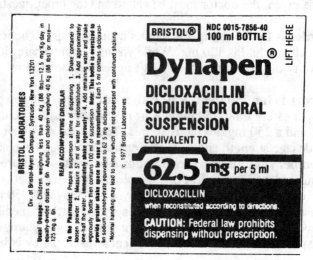

Figure 70

1. What is the recommended dosage in mg/kg/day? _____

2. What will the dosage be for this 32 kg child? _____

3. How many doses is this to be divided into? _____

4. How many mg per dose will this be? _____

5. If 125 mg is ordered q.6.h. is this a safe dosage? _____

ANSWERS **1.** 12.5 mg/kg/day   **2.** 400 mg/day   **3.** q.6.h. = 4 doses   **4.** 100 mg per dose   **5.** The 125 mg ordered is 25% more than the 100 mg per dose you calculated. Check with the doctor. It may be safe but it is on the high side.

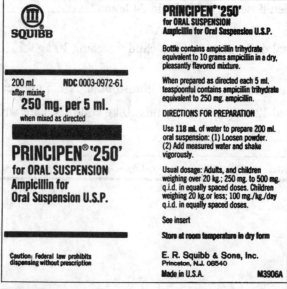

Figure 71

Refer to the ampicillin (Principen®) label in figure 71. Answer the following questions for a 12 lb infant.

1. What is the child's body weight in kg to the nearest tenth kg? _____

2. What is the recommended dosage in mg per day for this infant? _____

3. How many doses will this be divided into? _____

4. How many mg will this be per dose? _____

5. The order is to give 125 mg q.6.h. Is this safe? _____

6. How many mL would you need to administer a 125 mg dosage? _____

ANSWERS   **1.** 5 kg   **2.** 550 mg   **3.** 4 doses   **4.** 137.5 mg   **5.** Yes   **6.** 2.5 mL

A dosage of tetracycline 250 mg q.6.h. has been ordered for a child weighing 17 kg. Refer to the tetracycline label in figure 72 and determine if this is a safe dosage. Round body weight to the nearest whole lb.

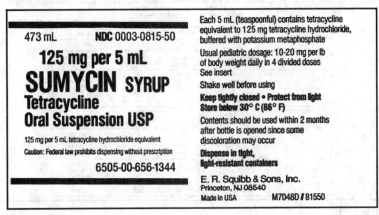

Figure 72

ANSWER   250 mg q.6.h. is an overdose for this child. 17 kg = 37 lb. This dosage range is 10–20 mg/lb/day. 10 mg × 37 lb = 370 mg; 20 mg × 37 lb = 740 mg. Four divided doses equal 370 mg ÷ 4 = 92.5 mg and 740 mg ÷ 4 = 185 mg per dose. The 250 mg per dose is too high. Notify the physician.

• DRUG INSERTS AND INFORMATION •

The labels you have just been reading are from oral syrups and suspensions, but the same calculation steps are necessary for dosages to be administered by the IV or IM route. Parenteral labels are much smaller in size and usually do not include dosage recommendations. To obtain these you will have to refer to the drug package inserts, the PDR, or other reference texts. Extensive details about each drug's chemistry, actions, adverse reactions, recommended administration, etc. is always included so it will be necessary for you to search for and select the information you need under the heading "Dosage and Administration." In the following exercises we have done the searching for you, and presented only those excerpts necessary for your calculations.

PROBLEM

Refer to the cefazolin (Kefzol®) label and information in figure 73 and answer the following questions.

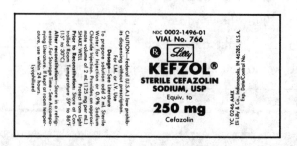

KEFZOL®, STERILE CEFAZOLIN SODIUM, USP

ADMINISTRATION AND DOSAGE

In children, a total daily dosage of 25 to 50 mg/kg (approximately 10 to 20 mg/lb) of body weight, divided into 3 or 4 equal doses, is effective for most mild to moderately severe infections (Table 5). Total daily dosage may be increased to 100 mg/kg (45 mg/lb) of body weight for severe infections.

TABLE 5. PEDIATRIC DOSAGE GUIDE

Weight		25 mg/kg/Day Divided into 3 Doses		25 mg/kg/Day Divided into 4 Doses	
lb	kg	Approximate Single Dose (mg q8h)	Vol (mL) Needed with Dilution of 125 mg/mL	Approximate Single Dose (mg q6h)	Vol (mL) Needed with Dilution of 125 mg/mL
10	4.5	40 mg	0.35 mL	30 mg	0.25 mL
20	9	75 mg	0.6 mL	55 mg	0.45 mL
30	13.6	115 mg	0.9 mL	85 mg	0.7 mL
40	18.1	150 mg	1.2 mL	115 mg	0.9 mL
50	22.7	190 mg	1.5 mL	140 mg	1.1 mL

Weight		50 mg/kg/Day Divided into 3 Doses		50 mg/kg/Day Divided into 4 Doses	
lb	kg	Approximate Single Dose (mg q8h)	Vol (mL) Needed with Dilution of 225 mg/mL	Approximate Single Dose (mg q6h)	Vol (mL) Needed with Dilution of 225 mg/mL
10	4.5	75 mg	0.35 mL	55 mg	0.25 mL
20	9	150 mg	0.7 mL	110 mg	0.5 mL
30	13.6	225 mg	1 mL	170 mg	0.75 mL
40	18.1	300 mg	1.35 mL	225 mg	1 mL
50	22.7	375 mg	1.7 mL	285 mg	1.25 mL

Figure 73

1. What is the dosage range in mg/kg/day for mild to moderate infections?

_____

2. What is the dosage range for mild to moderate infections in mg/lb/day?

_____

3. The total dosage will be divided into how many doses per day? _____

4. In severe infections what is the maximum dosage recommended in mg/kg

_____ mg/lb? _____

ANSWERS   **1.** 25 mg–50 mg   **2.** 10 mg–20 mg   **3.** 3–4 doses per day   **4.** 100 mg/kg; 45 mg/lb

If you examine Table 5 in this literature you will see that sample dosages are provided for several kg and lb weights, for both the 25 mg and 50 mg dosage, and for both 3 and 4 doses per day. Tables of this sort may be helpful, or harmful. They are helpful if they are easy to understand and the child whose dosage you are calculating fits exactly one of the weights listed; they are harmful if they tend to confuse, which is not uncommon. **The essential information that you need from the literature is 1. dosage range in mg/kg/day (or mg/lb/day); and 2. frequency of administration.** With this information you can quickly calculate what the dosages should be, and determine if the dosages ordered are correct.

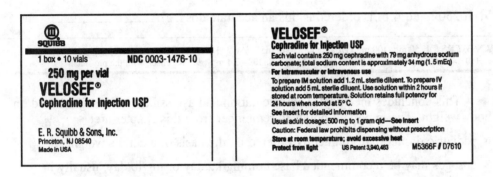

SQUIBB	VELOSEF®
1 box • 10 vials NDC 0003-1476-10	**Cephradine for Injection USP**
250 mg per vial	Each vial contains 250 mg cephradine with 79 mg anhydrous sodium carbonate; total sodium content is approximately 34 mg (1.5 mEq)
VELOSEF®	**For intramuscular or intravenous use**
Cephradine for Injection USP	To prepare IM solution add 1.2 mL sterile diluent. To prepare IV solution add 5 mL sterile diluent. Use solution within 2 hours if stored at room temperature. Solution retains full potency for 24 hours when stored at 5° C.
	See insert for detailed information
E. R. Squibb & Sons, Inc.	Usual adult dosage: 500 mg to 1 gram qid—See insert
Princeton, NJ 08540	Caution: Federal law prohibits dispensing without prescription
Made in USA	Store at room temperature; avoid excessive heat
	Protect from light US Patent 3,940,483 M5366F / D7610

VELOSEF® for INJECTION
Cephradine for Injection USP

DOSAGE AND ADMINISTRATION

Infants and Children
The usual dosage range of VELOSEF is 50 to 100 mg/kg/day (approximately 23 to 45 mg/lb/day) in equally divided doses four times a day and should be regulated by age, weight of the patient and severity of the infection being treated.

PEDIATRIC DOSAGE GUIDE				
	50 mg/kg/day		100 mg/kg/day	
Weight	Approx. single dose mg q6h	Volume needed @ 208 mg/mL dilution	Approx. single dose mg q6h	Volume needed @ 227 mg/mL dilution
lbs kg				
10 4.5	56 mg	0.27 mL	112 mg	0.5 mL
20 9.1	114 mg	0.55 mL	227 mg	1 mL
30 13.6	170 mg	0.82 mL	340 mg	1.5 mL
40 18.2	227 mg	1.1 mL	455 mg	2 mL
50 22.7	284 mg	1.4 mL	567 mg	2.5 mL

Figure 74

PROBLEM

Refer to the cephradine (Velosef®) label and literature in figure 74 and answer the following questions.

1. What is the usual dosage range in mg/kg/day? _____

2. What is the dosage range in mg/lb/day? _____

3. What is the recommended number of dosages per day? _____

4. What will the daily dosage range be for a child weighing 12 kg? _____

5. How many mg will be administered per dose? _____

6. If the order for this child is cephradine 250 mg q.6.h. is this an accurate dosage?

_____

7. What is the dosage range for a child weighing 19 lb? _____

8. What amount will be administered per dose? _____

9. If 250 mg q.6.h. is ordered is this an accurate dosage? _____

ANSWERS   1. 50 mg–100 mg/kg/day   **2.** 23–45 mg/lb/day   **3.** 4 doses per day   **4.** 600 mg–1200 mg
5. 150 mg–300 mg   **6.** Yes   **7.** 437 mg–855 mg   **8.** 109–214 mg   **9.** No, check with the physician

This concludes the chapter on calculation and assessment of dosages based on body weight. The important points to remember from this chapter are:

■ pediatric dosages are frequently ordered on the basis of a child's weight

■ dosages may be recommended based on mg/kg/day or mg/lb/day, usually in divided doses

■ body weight may need to be converted from kg to lb, or lb to kg to correlate with dosage recommendations

■ to convert lb to kg divide by 2.2

■ to convert kg to lb multiply by 2.2

■ calculating dosage is a two step procedure: first calculate the total daily dosage for the child's weight; then divide this by the number of doses to be administered

■ to check the accuracy of a doctor's order calculate the correct dosage for the child, then compare it with the dosage ordered

■ dosage discrepancies are much more critical if the dosage range is low, for example 4–6 mg, as opposed to high, for example 250 mg

■ factors that make discrepancies particularly dangerous are age, size, and overall medical condition of the child

■ if the drug label does not contain all the necessary information for safe administration, additional information should be obtained from the PDR, drug formularies, or the hospital pharmacist

SUMMARY SELF TEST
Dosage Calculation By Body Weight

DIRECTIONS   Read the dosage labels and literature provided and indicate if the following dosages are within normal safety limits. If they are not give the correct range. Express body weight conversions to the nearest tenth, and dosages to the nearest whole number.

PART I

1. Refer to the ticarcillin (Timentin®) label and literature and determine if a dosage of 1000 mg q.4.h. IV for a 52 lb child is correct. _____

2. Ticarcillin has also been ordered IV for a child weighing 32 lb. The dosage ordered is 1500 mg q.6.h. Is this a safe dosage? _____

3. A 45 lb child has an order for Ilosone® (erythromycin) oral susp. 250 mg q.6.h. Read the accompanying label and decide if this is a correct dosage.

_____

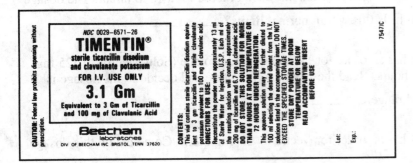

PART II

4. Zinacef® (cefuroxime) 375 mg has been ordered IV q.8.h. for a child weighing 44 lb. Determine if this is a safe dosage. _____

5. Zinacef® has also been ordered for a child weighing 84 lb. What would the dosage range be per day, and per dose if the medication is given q.6.h.?

_____

6. Oxacillin (Prostaphlin®) 250 mg q.6.h. p.o. has been ordered for a 44 lb child. Determine if this dosage is safe. _____

7. This same oral oxacillin solution has been ordered for a 16 lb infant. The dosage is 125 mg q.6.h. Is this within normal limits? _____

8. A 22 lb child has an order for IV methylprednisolone (Solu-Medrol®) 125 mg q.6.h. for 48 hours. Read the label and literature and decide if this dosage is within normal range. _____

9. A 7 kg infant has an order for Veetids® 125mg q.8.h. Comment on this dosage.

_____

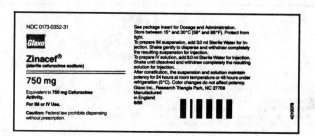

NDC 0173-0352-31

Glaxo

Zinacef®
(sterile cefuroxime sodium)

750 mg

Equivalent to 750 mg Cefuroxime Activity.

For IM or IV Use.

Caution: Federal law prohibits dispensing without prescription.

See package insert for Dosage and Administration. Store between 15° and 30°C (59° and 86°F). Protect from light.
To prepare IM suspension, add 3.0 ml Sterile Water for Injection. Shake gently to disperse and withdraw completely the resulting suspension for injection.
To prepare IV solution, add 8.0 ml Sterile Water for Injection. Shake until dissolved and withdraw completely the resulting solution for injection.
After constitution, the suspension and solution maintain potency for 24 hours at room temperature or 48 hours under refrigeration (5°C). Color changes do not affect potency.
Glaxo Inc., Research Triangle Park, NC 27709
Manufactured in England
6/88

ZINACEF®
[zin'ah-sef]
(sterile cefuroxime sodium, Glaxo)

DOSAGE AND ADMINISTRATION

Infants and Children Above 3 Months of Age: Administration of 50 to 100 mg/kg/day in equally divided doses every six to eight hours has been successful for most infections susceptible to cefuroxime. The higher dose of 100 mg/kg/day (not to exceed the maximum adult dose) should be used for the more severe or serious infections.
In bone and joint infections, 150 mg/kg/day (not to exceed the maximum adult dose) is recommended in equally divided doses every eight hours. In clinical trials a course of oral antibiotics was administered to children following the completion of parenteral administration of ZINACEF.
In cases of bacterial meningitis, larger doses of ZINACEF are recommended, 200 to 240 mg/kg/day intravenously in divided doses every six to eight hours.
In children with renal insufficiency, the frequency of dosage should be modified consistent with the recommendations for adults.

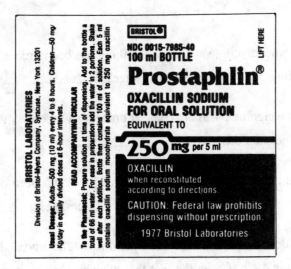

BRISTOL

NDC 0015-7985-40
100 ml BOTTLE

Prostaphlin®

LIFT HERE

OXACILLIN SODIUM
FOR ORAL SOLUTION
EQUIVALENT TO

250 mg per 5 ml

OXACILLIN
when reconstituted
according to directions.

CAUTION: Federal law prohibits
dispensing without prescription.

1977 Bristol Laboratories

BRISTOL LABORATORIES
Division of Bristol-Myers Company, Syracuse, New York 13201

Usual Dosage: Adults—500 mg (10 ml) every 4 to 6 hours. Children—50 mg/
Kg/day in equally divided doses at 6-hour intervals.

READ ACCOMPANYING CIRCULAR

To the Pharmacist: Prepare solution at time of dispensing. Add to the bottle a
total of 66 ml water. For ease in preparation add the water in 2 portions. Shake
well after each addition. Bottle then contains 100 ml of solution. Each 5 ml
contains oxacillin sodium monohydrate equivalent to 250 mg oxacillin.

NDC 0009-0190-09
2 ml Act-O-Vial®

Solu-Medrol® 125 mg*
Sterile Powder

methylprednisolone sodium
succinate for injection, USP

For IV or IM use
See package insert for complete product
information.

Each 2 ml (when mixed) contains:
*methylprednisolone sodium succinate equiv.
to methylprednisolone, 125 mg.
Lyophilized in container   812 993 202
The Upjohn Company
Kalamazoo, Michigan 49001, USA

SOLU–MEDROL®
brand of methylprednisolone sodium succinate sterile
powder
(methylprednisolone sodium succinate for
injection, USP)
For Intravenous or Intramuscular
Administration

DOSAGE AND ADMINISTRATION
When high dose therapy is desired, the recommended dose of
SOLU-MEDROL Sterile Powder (methylprednisolone sodium succinate) is 30 mg/kg administered intravenously
over at least 30 minutes. This dose may be repeated every 4
to 6 hours for 48 hours.

Dosage may be reduced for infants and children but should
be governed more by the severity of the condition and response of the patient than by age or size. It should not be less
than 0.5 mg per kg every 24 hours.

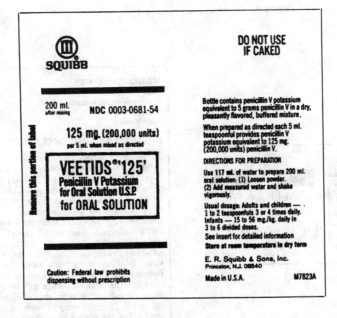

SQUIBB

DO NOT USE
IF CAKED

200 ml.
after mixing   NDC 0003-0681-54

125 mg. (200,000 units)
per 5 ml. when mixed as directed

VEETIDS®'125'
Penicillin V Potassium
for Oral Solution U.S.P.
for ORAL SOLUTION

Remove this portion of label

Caution: Federal law prohibits
dispensing without prescription

Bottle contains penicillin V potassium
equivalent to 5 grams penicillin V in a dry,
pleasantly flavored, buffered mixture.

When prepared as directed each 5 ml.
teaspoonful provides penicillin V
potassium equivalent to 125 mg.
(200,000 units) penicillin V.

DIRECTIONS FOR PREPARATION

Use 117 ml. of water to prepare 200 ml.
oral solution: (1) Loosen powder.
(2) Add measured water and shake
vigorously.

Usual dosage: Adults and children —
1 to 2 teaspoonfuls 3 or 4 times daily.
Infants — 15 to 56 mg./kg. daily in
3 to 6 divided doses.

See insert for detailed information
Store at room temperature in dry form

E. R. Squibb & Sons, Inc.
Princeton, N.J. 08540

Made in U.S.A.   M7823A

PART III

10. A dosage of vancomycin (Vancocin®) 100 mg has been ordered q.6.h. IV for a child weighing 22 lb. Is this a safe dosage? _____

11. Another child weighing 54 lb also has an order for vancomycin IV. Determine what the dosage should be q.6.h. _____

12. Amoxil® oral amoxicillin suspension 125 mg q.8.h. has been ordered for an infant weighing 14 lb. Determine if this is a safe dosage? _____

13. Calculate the dosage range per day and per dose of the amoxicillin oral susp. for a child weighing 41 lb. Given the fact that this child has a severe infection, and that the dosage of the solution is 250 mg per 5 mL, what would you expect the order to be q.8.h? _____

14. A child weighing 30 kg has an order for cephapirin (Cefadyl®) 60 mg IV q.4.h. Read the literature and decide if this dosage is correct. _____

15. A 46 lb child has a dosage of oral hetacillin 112.5 mg ordered q.6.h. Notice that the dosage on this Versapen® label is specified per dose, not per day. Calculate to determine if the dosage is within normal range. _____

16. An infant weighing 17 lb also has an order for hetacillin p.o. The dosage ordered is 45 mg q.6.h. Is this a normal dose? How many mL would you administer to give the correct dosage? _____

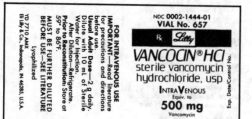

VANCOCIN® HCl
[văn ′kō-sĭn ăch ′sē-ĕl]
(vancomycin hydrochloride)
Sterile, USP
IntraVenous

DOSAGE AND ADMINISTRATION

Patients with Normal Renal Function
Adults —The usual daily intravenous dose is 2 g divided either as 500 mg every 6 hours or 1 g every 12 hours. Each dose should be administered over a period of at least 60 minutes. Other patient factors, such as age or obesity, may call for modification of the usual daily dose.
Children —The total daily intravenous dosage of Vancocin® HCl (vancomycin hydrochloride, Lilly), calculated on the basis of 40 mg/kg of body weight, can be divided and incorporated into the child's 24-hour fluid requirement. Each dose should be administered over a period of at least 60 minutes.
Infants and Neonates —In neonates and young infants, the total daily intravenous dosage may be lower. In both neonates and infants, an initial dose of 15 mg/kg is suggested, followed by 10 mg/kg every 12 hours for neonates in the first week of life and every 8 hours thereafter up to the age of 1 month. Close monitoring of serum concentrations of vancomycin may be warranted in these patients.

AMOXIL®

amoxicillin
for oral suspension

NDC 0029–6009–22
Equivalent to
7.50 Gm Amoxicillin

When reconstituted
each 5 ml will contain
250 mg
Amoxicillin
as the trihydrate
150 ml

Beecham
laboratories

9405820

DIRECTIONS FOR MIXING:
Tap bottle until all powder flows freely. Add approximately 1/3 of the total amount of water for reconstitution (total = 111 ml) and shake vigorously to wet powder. Add the remainder of the water and again shake vigorously. Each 5 ml (1 teaspoonful) will then contain Amoxicillin Trihydrate equivalent to 250 mg Amoxicillin

USUAL DOSAGE:
Adults: 250 mg–500 mg every 8 hours –
Children: 20–40 mg/day in divided doses every 8 hours – depending on age, weight and severity of infection.

READ ACCOMPANYING INSERT BEFORE USE

U.S. PATENT 3,192,198 & RE. 28,744

T82

NDC 0015-7827-28
Cefadyl®
STERILE CEPHAPIRIN
SODIUM FOR I.M. OR I.V. USE
EQUIVALENT TO
500 mg
CEPHAPIRIN

BRISTOL LABORATORIES
Div. of Bristol-Myers Company
Syracuse, New York 13201

This vial contains cephapirin sodium equivalent to 500 mg cephapirin. **Usual Dosage: Adults**—500 mg to 1 g, 6h.
For I.M. use, add 1 ml Sterile or Bacteriostatic Water for Injection, U.S.P. Each 1.2 ml contains 500 mg of cephapirin.
For I.V. use, add 10 ml Sterile or Bacteriostatic Water for Injection, U.S.P. Each ml contains 50 mg of cephapirin.
Following reconstitution, the solution is stable for 12 hours at room temperature or 10 days under refrigeration.
READ ACCOMPANYING CIRCULAR for detailed indications, dosage and precautions.
CAUTION: Federal law prohibits dispensing without prescription.
© 1977 Bristol Laboratories
7827280RL-01

CEFADYL®
(sterile cephapirin sodium)
Dosage and Administration:

Children—The dosage is in accordance with age, weight, and severity of infection. The recommended total daily dose is 40 to 80 mg/Kg (20 to 40 mg/lb) administered in four equally divided doses. The drug has not been extensively studied in infants, therefore, in the treatment of children under the age of three months the relative benefit/risk should be considered.

BRISTOL™

NDC 0015-7808-40
100 ml. Bottle

VERSAPEN®
HETACILLIN

FOR ORAL SUSPENSION

EQUIVALENT TO
112.5 mg.
per 5 ml.
AMPICILLIN

when reconstituted
according to directions.

CAUTION: Federal law prohibits dispensing without prescription.

BRISTOL LABORATORIES
Div. of Bristol-Myers Company
Syracuse, New York 13201

Usual Dosage:
Patients weighing 88 lbs. (40 Kg.) or more—225 mg. q.i.d. Patients weighing less than 88 lbs. (40 Kg.)—2.5 mg./lb. q.i.d.

READ ACCOMPANYING CIRCULAR

To the Pharmacist: Prepare suspension at time of dispensing. Add 73 ml. water to the bottle and shake well. This provides 100 ml. of suspension.

LIFT HERE

PART IV

17. A child weighing 15 kg with a diagnosis of bacterial meningitis has an order for cefuroxome (Kefurox®) 750 mg IV q.6.h. From the available information calculate to determine if this is a correct dosage. _____

18. An infant suffering from a genitourinary tract infection has an order for IV ampicillin (Omnipen-N®) 125 mg q.6.h. The child weighs 12 lb. Is this a correct dosage? _____

19. A 14 lb infant has ampicillin ordered for a respiratory infection. The doctor has ordered 62.5 mg IV q.6.h. Comment on this dosage. _____

20. Ceftazidime (Tazidime®) 1250 mg IV is ordered q.8.h. for a child weighing 55 lb. After reviewing the literature determine if this is a safe dosage. _____

Wyeth
Omnipen®-N
(ampicillin sodium)
Injection
equivalent to
125 mg ampicillin per vial
for **IM** or **IV** use

NDC 0008-0315-01
Single-dose vial containing Omnipen-N equivalent to 125 mg ampicillin per vial when reconstituted with 1 ml (for IM use) or 5 ml (for IV use) Sterile Water for Injection, USP, or Bacteriostatic Water for Injection, USP (TUBEX®).
Use solution within 1 hour
Made and printed in USA   U0315-01-1
WYETH LABORATORIES INC.
Philadelphia, PA 19101

Wyeth®
Omnipen®-N
(ampicillin sodium)
For Parenteral Administration

Dosage (IM or IV)

Infection	Organisms	Adults	Children*
Respiratory tract	streptococci, pneumococci, nonpenicillinase-producing staphylococci, H. influenzae	250-500 mg q. 6 h.	25-50 mg/kg/day in equal doses q. 6 h.
Gastrointestinal tract	susceptible pathogens	500 mg q. 6 h.	50 mg/kg/day in equal doses q. 6 h.
Genitourinary tract	susceptible gram-negative or gram-positive pathogens	500 mg q. 6 h.	50 mg/kg/day in equal doses q. 6 h.
Urethritis (acute) in adult males	N. gonorrhoeae	500 mg b.i.d. for 1 day (IM)	
	(In complications such as prostatitis and epididymitis, prolonged and intensive therapy is recommended. Gonorrhea cases with suspected primary lesion of syphilis should have dark-field examinations before treatment. In any case suspected of concomitant syphilis, monthly serologic tests for at least 4 months are necessary.)		
Bacterial meningitis	N. meningitidis, H. influenzae	8-14 gram/day	100-200 mg/kg/day
	(Initial treatment is usually by IV drip, followed by frequent [q. 3-4 h.] IM injections.) S. viridans		

*Children's dosage recommendations are intended for those whose weight will not result in a dosage higher than for the adult.

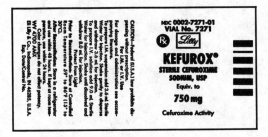

KEFUROX™

[kĕf'ōō-rŏcks]
sterile cefuroxime sodium)

DOSAGE AND ADMINISTRATION

Infants and Children Above 3 Months of Age—Administration of 50 to 100 mg/kg/day in equally divided doses every 6 to 8 hours has been successful for most infections susceptible to cefuroxime. The higher dose of 100 mg/kg/day (not to exceed the maximum adult dose) should be used for the more severe or serious infections.

In cases of bacterial meningitis, larger doses of Kefurox are recommended, initially 200 to 240 mg/kg/day intravenously in divided doses every 6 to 8 hours.

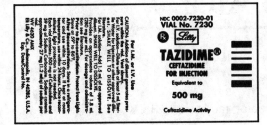

TAZIDIME™

[tă'zĭ-dēm]
(ceftazidime)
for injection

DOSAGE AND ADMINISTRATION

The guidelines for dosage of Tazidime™ (ceftazidime, Lilly) are listed in Table 3. The following dosage schedule is recommended:

Table 3: Recommended Dosage Schedule for Ceftazidime

	Dose	Frequency
Adults		
Usual recommended dose	**1 g IV or IM**	**q8 or 12h**
Uncomplicated urinary tract infections	250 mg IV or IM	q12h
Bone and joint infections	2 g IV	q12h
Complicated urinary tract infections	500 mg IV or IM	q8 or 12h
Uncomplicated pneumonia; mild skin and skin-structure infections	500 mg–1 g IV or IM	q8h
Serious gynecologic and intra-abdominal infections	2 g IV	q8h
Meningitis	2 g IV	q8h
Very severe life-threatening infections, especially in immunocompromised patients	2 g IV	q8h
Pseudomonal lung infections in patients with cystic fibrosis with normal renal function*	30–50 mg/kg IV to a maximum of 6 g/day	q8h
Neonates (0–4 weeks)	30 mg/kg IV	q12h
Infants and Children (1 month to 12 years)	30–50 mg/kg IV to a maximum of 6 g/day†	q8h

ANSWERS

1. Yes   **2.** No. Too high. 725 mg–1088 mg/dose is average   **3.** Yes   **4.** Yes   **5.** 1910–3820 mg/day; 478–955 mg/dose   **6.** Yes
7. No. Normal is 91 mg/dose   **8.** Yes   **9.** Within normal range of 35–131 mg/dose   **10.** Yes   **11.** 245 mg   **12.** Not safe. 43–85 mg/dose is average   **13.** Dosage would be 250 mg q.8.h.   Range: 372–744 mg/day; 124–248 mg/dose   **14.** Not correct. Range is 1200–2400 mg/day in four doses (q.6.h.) not six doses (q.4.h.) ordered. Correct dosage is 300–600 mg q.6.h.   **15.** Yes   **16.** Yes; 2 mL = 45 mg   **17.** Yes   **18.** No. 69 mg/dose is normal   **19.** Within normal range of 40–80 mg/dose   **20.** Yes

19
Pediatric Dosage Calculation by Body Surface Area

OBJECTIVES
The student will
1. determine BSA's using the West Nomogram
2. calculate dosages using BSA
3. assess the accuracy of dosages prescribed on the basis of BSA

INTRODUCTION
A child's body surface area is determined by comparing his/her weight and height with averages or norms, on a graph called a nomogram. A number of drugs are prescribed on the basis of BSA, particularly antineoplastic drugs, and there is some indication that BSA may see increasing use in other drug categories as well. This method of dosage calculation is considered by some authorities to be more accurate than the previously discussed body weight method, since BSA correlates the child's size with his/her physiological development, and ability to tolerate specific drugs. The nursing responsibility for checking dosages based on BSA varies widely among hospitals, therefore this chapter will cover all three essentials: calculation of BSA, calculation of dosages based on BSA, and assessment of physician orders based on BSA.

• CALCULATION OF BSA •

The BSA is determined by using a child's weight, height, and a nomogram such as the West nomogram in figure 75. If the child is of roughly normal height and weight for his or her age the BSA can be determined from weight alone. If you refer to the enclosed column second from the left on the nomogram you can see, for example, that a child weighing 30 lb has a BSA of 0.60 M².

Before we move on to having you determine some BSA's on your own, we need to point out a peculiarity of nomograms that could cause confusion. Notice that neither the calibrations nor the numbers identifying them rise consistently from the bottom to the top of the graph. **To identify the correct values you must first read the numbers, then determine what the calibrations between them are measuring.** Refer to the weight—M² column second from the left again, and notice that there is a very large space between 2 and 3 lb, while at the top of the scale there is a very narrow space between 80 and 90 lb. Between 15 and 20 lb there are 1 lb increments in calibration representing 16, 17, 18, and 19 lb, but between 80 and 90 lb only one calibration, which represents 85 lb. Similarly, on the bottom of the M² scale there are four calibrations between 0.10 and 0.15, which represent 0.11, 0.12, 0.13, and 0.14 M². On the top of the M² scale there is only one calibration between 1.20 and 1.30 which represents 1.25 M². So once again look at the numbers and calibrations very carefully to determine what the measurements are.

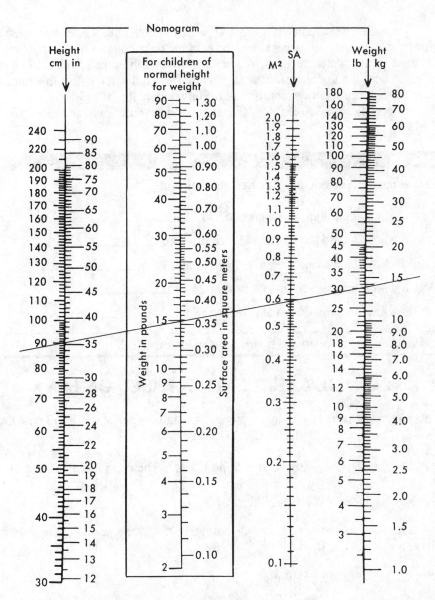

Figure 75. West Nomogram. From Behman, R.E. and Vaughan, V.C. Nelson Textbook of Pediatrics, 12th edition. Philadelphia, W.B. Saunders Co. 1987. Reprinted by permission.

PROBLEM

Read the nomogram provided and indicate the BSA in M² for the following children of normal height and weight.

1. A child weighing 24 lb _____

2. A child weighing 42 lb _____

3. A child weighing 11 lb _____

4. A child weighing 52 lb _____

5. A child weighing 75 lb _____

ANSWERS   **1.** 0.50 M²   **2.** 0.78 M²   **3.** 0.29 M²   **4.** 0.90 M²   **5.** 1.15 M²

BSA can also be calculated using both weight and height. The extreme left column for height (in cm and inches), and the extreme right column for weight (in lb and kg) are used for this determination. A ruler is placed on the graph from the height to the weight column, and the surface area (SA) in M² is indicated where this line intersects the SA column second from the right. For example the line already on the nomogram identifies a BSA of 0.59 M² for a child weighing 30 lb and measuring 35 inches.

PROBLEM

Use the nomogram provided to calculate the following BSA's.

1. The child is 100 cm long and weighs 55 lb _____

2. A child whose length is 120 cm and weight 40 kg _____

3. A child whose height and weight are 65 cm and 13 kg _____

4. A child whose height is 58 in and weight 12 kg _____

5. A child whose length is 45 in and weight 18 lb _____

ANSWERS   **1.** 0.86 M²   **2.** 1.2 M²   **3.** 0.51 M²   **4.** 0.66 M²   **5.** 0.49 M²

• DOSAGE CALCULATION BASED ON BSA •

A number of drugs specify children's dosages in mg or u per M². If you know the child's BSA, dosage calculation is simple multiplication.

EXAMPLE 1   Dosage recommended is 5 mg per M². The child has a BSA of 1.1 M².

1.1×5 mg = **5.5 mg**

EXAMPLE 2   The recommended child's dosage is 25–50 mg per M². The child has a BSA of 0.76 M².

$0.76 \times 25 = 19$ mg

$0.76 \times 50 = 38$ mg

The dosage range is **19–38 mg**

If a drug recommends dosages only for adults a formula is used to calculate the child's dose. The formula uses the average adult dose, the average adult BSA (1.7 M²), and the child's BSA in M².

FORMULA:

$$\text{Dosage} = \frac{\text{Child's BSA}}{1.7 \text{ M}^2} \times \text{Adult Dose}$$

EXAMPLE 1   The doctor has ordered an antibiotic whose average adult dose is 250 mg. What will the dose be for a child with a BSA of 0.41 M²?

$$\frac{0.41}{1.7} \times 250 \text{ mg} = \textbf{60.3 mg}$$

EXAMPLE 2   The normal adult dosage of a drug is 1000 u. What will the dosage be for a child whose BSA is 0.56 M²?

$$\frac{0.56}{1.7} \times 1000 \text{ u} = \textbf{329.4 u}$$

PROBLEM

Determine the child's dosage for the following drugs. Express answers to the nearest tenth.

1. The adult dose of a drug is 5–10 mg. What will the dosage range be for a child whose BSA is 0.36 M²? _____

2. A child with a BSA of 1.15 M² has an order for a drug whose adult dose is 750 mg. What should the dosage be? _____

3. The average adult dose of an antibiotic is 500 mg. What will the dosage be for a child with a BSA of 0.62 M²? _____

4. The doctor has ordered a dosage of 7 mg of a drug for a child with a BSA of 0.47 M². The average adult dose is 25 mg. Is this a correct dosage? _____

5. A dose of 42 u of a drug has been ordered for a child with a BSA of 0.72 M². The average adult dose is 100 mg. Is this dosage correct? _____

ANSWERS   **1.** 1.1 to 2.2 mg   **2.** 507.4 mg   **3.** 182.4 mg   **4.** Yes   **5.** Yes

This concludes dosage calculations based on a child's BSA. The important points to remember from this chapter are:

■ BSA is determined from a graph called a nomogram, using the child's height and weight

■ BSA correlates physiological development and size and is considered by some to be more accurate than body weight calculations

■ reading a nomogram requires particular care because neither the calibrations nor incremental numbers rise consistently on the chart from bottom to top

■ when dosage recommendations for children specify mg/M², calculating the dosage is simple multiplication

■ when dosages are specified only for adults a formula is used to calculate a child's dosage from the adult dose

■ to determine if a doctor's order is correct, calculate the child's dose from the BSA in M², then compare with the dosage ordered

Pediatric Dosage Calculation By BSA

DIRECTIONS Calculate the following child's dosages. When a physician order is given, determine if it is correct. If the order is incorrect give the normal dosage. Express answers to the nearest tenth.

1. The recommended child's dosage is 5–10 mg/M². The child's BSA is 0.43 M².
_____

2. A dosage of 500 mg has been ordered for a child with a BSA of 1.7 M². The recommended adult dosage is 500 mg. Is this dosage correct? _____

3. The adult dose of a drug is 300 mg. Calculate the dosage for a child with a BSA of 0.64 M². _____

4. The average adult dose is 750 mg. Calculate the dose a child with a BSA of 1.4 M² should receive. _____

5. A drug with a normal adult dose of 15 mg has been ordered for a child with a BSA of 0.6 M² in a dosage of 5 mg. _____

6. The recommended child's dosage is 40 mg/M². The child has a BSA of 0.81 M². _____

7. A dosage of 26 u of a drug whose adult dose is 60 u has been ordered for a child with a BSA of 0.44 M². _____

8. The average adult dose of a drug is 75 to 100 mg. A dosage of 60 mg has been ordered for a child with a BSA of 1.2 M². _____

9. The drug has an adult dosage of 1 g. The child's BSA is 0.47 M². _____

10. A child with a BSA of 0.86 M² has an order of 20 mg for a drug with an average adult dose of 40 mg. _____

11. A child with a BSA of 0.96 M² has an order for 23 u of a drug whose adult dose is 40 u. _____

12. A dosage of 4 mg of a drug with an adult range of 10–15 mg has been ordered for a child with a BSA of 0.98 M². _____

13. An IV drug has an adult dose of 10–20 mg. A child with a BSA of 0.74 M² has an order for 10 mg. _____

14. An antibiotic whose adult dose is 80 mg has been ordered for a child with a BSA of 0.5 M². Calculate if the 24 mg dose ordered is within normal range.

   _____

15. A dosage of 31 mg of a drug has been ordered for a child with a BSA of 0.88 M². The adult dose is 60 mg. _____

16. A child with a BSA of 0.82 M² has been ordered to receive 20 mg of a drug whose adult dose is 75 mg. _____

17. A child with a BSA of 0.74 M² is to receive a drug with an adult dosage of 300,000 u. What should his dose be? _____

18. A child with a BSA of 0.31 M² has an order for 40 mg of a drug with a recommended adult range of 200–300 mg. Is this the correct dose? _____

19. A child with a BSA of 0.78 M² has an order for 184 mg of a drug whose adult dose is 400 mg. _____

20. A drug has been ordered for a child whose BSA is 0.92 M². The average adult dose is 10 mg. Calculate if the 5 mg dosage ordered is correct. _____

21. A dosage of 26 mg has been ordered of an antibiotic drug whose normal adult dose is 75 mg. The child's BSA is 0.59 M². Is this dosage correct?

   _____

22. A child with a BSA of 1.42 M² is to receive a drug with a recommended adult dose of 125 mg. _____

23. A child with a BSA of 0.74 M² has an order for 20 mg of an IV drug. The adult dose is 45 mg. _____

24. A dosage of 7 u of a drug has been ordered for a child with a BSA of 0.38 M². The adult dose is 30 u. _____

25. A child with a BSA of 1 M² has an order for 150 mg of a drug which has an adult average dose of 200 mg. _____

26. Calculate the dosage of a drug with a recommended child's dosage of 20 mg/M² for a child with a BSA of 0.50 M². _____

27. An antibiotic with a normal adult dose of 150 mg has been ordered for a child whose BSA is 0.7 M². The dose ordered is 62 mg. _____

28. A dosage of 14 mg of an IV drug has been ordered for a child whose BSA is 0.68 M². Is this correct if the normal adult dose is 35 mg? _____

29. A dosage of 66 mg has been ordered for a child with a BSA of 0.9 M². The adult dose is 125 mg. _____

30. A dosage of 6 mg of a drug has been ordered for a child with a BSA of 0.53 M². The adult dose is 20 mg. _____

ANSWERS

1. 2.2–4.3 mg   2. Yes   3. 112.9 mg   4. 617.6 mg   5. Correct   6. 32.4 mg   7. Too high; 15.5 u normal   8. Correct   9. 276.5 mg   10. Correct   11. Correct   12. Too low; average 5.8–8.6 mg   13. Too high; 4.4–8.7 mg   14. Normal   15. Correct   16. Too low; 36.2 mg normal   17. 130,588.2 u   18. Yes   19. Correct   20. Correct   21. Correct   22. 104.4 mg   23. Correct   24. Correct   25. Too high; 117.6 mg normal   26. 10 mg   27. Correct   28. Yes   29. Correct   30. Correct

20
Pediatric Oral and Parenteral Medications

OBJECTIVES
The student will
1. explain how suspensions are measured and administered
2. list the precautions of IM and s.c. injection in infants and children
3. calculate pediatric oral dosages
4. calculate pediatric IM and s.c. dosages

INTRODUCTION
Two differences between adult and pediatric dosages will be immediately apparent: **most oral drugs are prepared as liquids** because infants and small children cannot be expected to swallow tablets easily, if at all, and **dosages are dramatically smaller**. The oral route is used whenever possible, but when a child cannot swallow, or the drug is ineffective given orally, drugs will be administered by a parenteral route.

Both the subcutaneous and intramuscular routes may be used depending on the type of drug to be administered. The small muscle size of infants and children limits the use of the intramuscular route, as does the nature of the drug being used. For example, most antibiotics are administered intravenously rather than intramuscularly.

• ORAL MEDICATIONS •

Most oral pediatric drugs are prepared as liquids to facilitate ease in swallowing. If the child is old enough to cooperate these dosages may be measured in a medication cup. Solutions may also be measured using oral syringes, such as the one shown in figure 76. Oral syringes are calibrated the same as hypodermic syringes, with the addition of household measures, for example tsp. They are frequently amber colored and have different sized tips to prevent accidental use with hypodermic needles. On some oral syringes the tip is positioned off center (termed eccentric), to further distinguish them from hypodermic syringes. If oral syringes are not available hypodermic syringes (**without the needle**) can also be used for dosage measurement. In addition to accuracy syringes provide an excellent method of administering oral liquid drugs to infants and small children.

When volumes are extremely small oral liquids are measured using a calibrated medication dropper which is an integral part of the medication bottle. These may be calibrated in mL, like the dropper shown in figure 77, or in actual drug weights, for example 25 mg, or 50 mg.

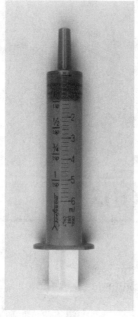

Figure 76

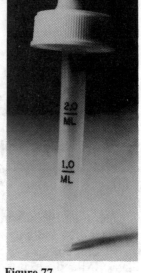

Figure 77

Care must be taken with oral liquid drugs to identify those prepared as **suspensions**. A suspension consists of an insoluable drug in a liquid base, as for example in the amoxicillin preparation in figure 78. The drug in a suspension settles to the bottom of the bottle between uses, and **thorough mixing immediately prior to pouring is mandatory**. Suspensions must also be administered to the child immediately after measurement to prevent the drug settling out again, and an incomplete dosage being administered.

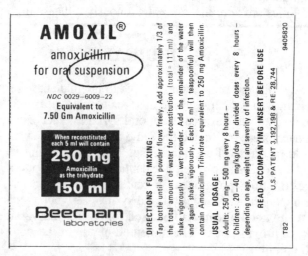

Figure 78

When a tablet or capsule is administered the child's mouth must be checked to be certain it has actually been swallowed. If swallowing is a problem some tablets can be crushed and given in a small amount of applesauce, ice cream or juice if the child has no dietary restrictions which would contraindicate this. Keep in mind, however, that **enteric coated and timed release tablets or capsules cannot be crushed** since this would destroy the coating which allows them to function on a delayed action basis.

• PARENTERAL MEDICATIONS •

The drugs given the most often via the subcutaneous route are insulin, and immunizations which specifically require the subcutaneous route. Any site with sufficient subcutaneous tissue may be used, with the upper arm being the site of choice for immunizations. The intramuscular route is used most frequently for preoperative and postoperative medications for sedation and pain, and for immunizations such as DPT (diphtheria, pertussis, tetanus) which must be administered deep IM. The intramuscular site of choice for infants and small children is the vastus lateralis or rectus femoris of the thigh, because the gluteal muscles do not develop until a child has learned to walk. Usually not more than 1 mL is injected per site, and sites are rotated regularly.

Dosage calculation is the same as for adults, except **dosages are usually calculated to the nearest hundredth, and measured using a tuberculin syringe**. (Refer to Chapter 10 if you need to review the calibrations and use of a TB syringe). There is less margin for error in pediatric dosages, and calculations and measurements are routinely double checked.

This concludes the chapter on pediatric oral and parenteral medication administration. The important points to remember are:

- care must be taken when administering oral drugs to be positive the child has actually swallowed the dosage

- if liquid medications are prepared as suspensions, mix thoroughly prior to measurement, and administer immediately

- the IM site of choice for infants and children is the vastus lateralis or rectus femoris of the thigh

- usually not more than 1 mL is injected per IM or s.c. site and sites are rotated regularly

- pediatric dosages are usually calculated to the nearest hundredth and measured using a TB syringe

SUMMARY SELF TEST
Pediatric Oral And Parenteral Medications

DIRECTIONS Use the labels provided to measure the following oral dosages.

PART I

1. Prepare a 375 mg dosage of oxacillin. _____

2. Prepare a 250 mg dosage of amoxicillin. _____

3. A dosage of Mycostatin® 150,000 u has been ordered. _____

4. What special precaution is necessary when preparing this Mycostatin® medication? _____

5. Prepare a 60 mg dosage of theophylline. _____

6. A dosage of penicillin V potassium 400,000 u has been ordered.

_____

7. A 10 mg dosage of dioctyl sodium sulfosuccinate has been ordered.

_____

8. Tempra® 0.6 mL has been ordered. The bottle has a calibrated medicine dropper. _____

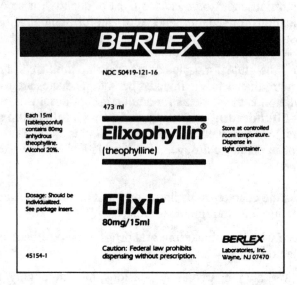

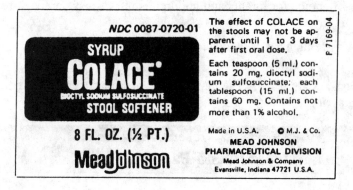

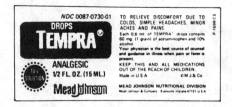

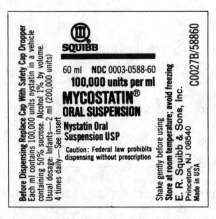

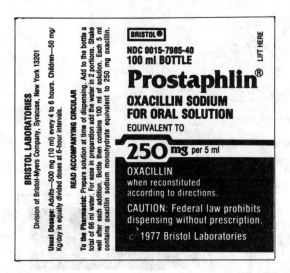

BRISTOL LABORATORIES
Division of Bristol-Myers Company, Syracuse, New York 13201

Usual Dosage: Adults—500 mg (10 ml) every 4 to 6 hours. Children—50 mg/Kg/day in equally divided doses at 6-hour intervals.

READ ACCOMPANYING CIRCULAR

To the Pharmacist: Prepare solution at time of dispensing. Add to the bottle a total of 66 ml water. For ease in preparation add the water in 2 portions. Shake well after each addition. Bottle then contains 100 ml of solution. Each 5 ml contains oxacillin sodium monohydrate equivalent to 250 mg oxacillin.

LIFT HERE

BRISTOL®
NDC 0015-7985-40
100 ml BOTTLE
Prostaphlin®
OXACILLIN SODIUM
FOR ORAL SOLUTION
EQUIVALENT TO
250 mg per 5 ml
OXACILLIN
when reconstituted
according to directions.
CAUTION: Federal law prohibits
dispensing without prescription.
© 1977 Bristol Laboratories

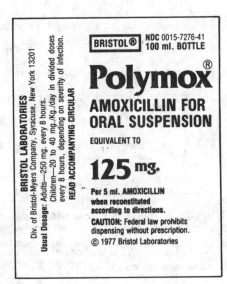

BRISTOL LABORATORIES
Div. of Bristol-Myers Company, Syracuse, New York 13201

Usual Dosage: Adults—250 mg. every 8 hours.
Children—20 to 40 mg./Kg./day in divided doses every 8 hours, depending on severity of infection.
READ ACCOMPANYING CIRCULAR

BRISTOL® NDC 0015-7276-41
100 ml. BOTTLE
Polymox®
AMOXICILLIN FOR
ORAL SUSPENSION
EQUIVALENT TO
125 mg.
Per 5 ml. AMOXICILLIN
when reconstituted
according to directions.
CAUTION: Federal law prohibits
dispensing without prescription.
© 1977 Bristol Laboratories

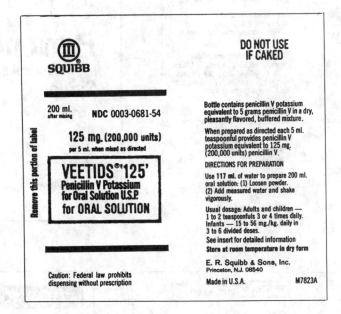

SQUIBB

200 ml.
after mixing   NDC 0003-0681-54

125 mg. (200,000 units)
per 5 ml. when mixed as directed

VEETIDS®'125'
Penicillin V Potassium
for Oral Solution U.S.P.
for ORAL SOLUTION

Remove this portion of label

Caution: Federal law prohibits
dispensing without prescription

**DO NOT USE
IF CAKED**

Bottle contains penicillin V potassium
equivalent to 5 grams penicillin V in a dry,
pleasantly flavored, buffered mixture.

When prepared as directed each 5 ml.
teaspoonful provides penicillin V
potassium equivalent to 125 mg.
(200,000 units) penicillin V.

DIRECTIONS FOR PREPARATION

Use 117 ml. of water to prepare 200 ml.
oral solution: (1) Loosen powder.
(2) Add measured water and shake
vigorously.

Usual dosage: Adults and children —
1 to 2 teaspoonfuls 3 or 4 times daily.
Infants — 15 to 56 mg./kg. daily in
3 to 6 divided doses.
See insert for detailed information
Store at room temperature in dry form

E. R. Squibb & Sons, Inc.
Princeton, N.J. 08540

Made in U.S.A.   M7823A

PART II

9. A bottle of Principen® "250" is available in the powdered form. Read the label and locate the type and amount of solution necessary to reconstitute this drug.

_____

10. What will the dosage strength of the reconstituted medication be?

_____

11. Prepare a 300 mg dosage of Principen®. _____

12. Prepare a 225 mg dosage of hetacillin. _____

13. A 100 mg dosage of clindamycin is ordered. _____

14. Prepare a dosage of dicloxacillin 125 mg. _____

15. Prepare a 4 mg dosage of Proventil®. _____

16. Prepare a 300 mg dosage of erythromycin. _____

17. A dosage of amoxicillin 60 mg has been ordered. _____

SQUIBB

200 ml.   NDC 0003-0972-61
after mixing
250 mg. per 5 ml.
when mixed as directed

PRINCIPEN® '250'
for ORAL SUSPENSION
Ampicillin for
Oral Suspension U.S.P.

Caution: Federal law prohibits
dispensing without prescription

PRINCIPEN® '250'
for ORAL SUSPENSION
Ampicillin for Oral Suspension U.S.P.

Bottle contains ampicillin trihydrate
equivalent to 10 grams ampicillin in a dry,
pleasantly flavored mixture.

When prepared as directed each 5 ml.
teaspoonful contains ampicillin trihydrate
equivalent to 250 mg. ampicillin.

DIRECTIONS FOR PREPARATION

Use 118 ml. of water to prepare 200 ml.
oral suspension: (1) Loosen powder.
(2) Add measured water and shake
vigorously.

Usual dosage: Adults, and children
weighing over 20 kg.; 250 mg. to 500 mg.
q.i.d. in equally spaced doses. Children
weighing 20 kg. or less; 100 mg./kg./day
q.i.d. in equally spaced doses.

See insert

Store at room temperature in dry form

E. R. Squibb & Sons, Inc.
Princeton, N.J. 08540
Made in U.S.A.   M3906A

SCHERING

NDC-0085-0315-02

16 fl. oz. (1 pint)

Proventil®
brand of albuterol sulfate
Syrup

2
mg*

per 5 ml

*Potency expressed
as albuterol.

BRISTOL LABORATORIES
Div of Bristol-Myers Company Syracuse, New York 13201

Usual Dosage: Children weighing less than 40 Kg (88 lbs)—12.5 mg Kg day in
equally-divided doses q 6h Adults and children weighing 40 Kg (88 lbs) or more—
125 mg q 6h

READ ACCOMPANYING CIRCULAR

To the Pharmacist: Prepare suspension at time of dispensing 1. Shake container to
loosen powder 2. Measure 57 ml of water for reconstitution 3. Add approximately
one-half the water; **immediately shake vigorously** * 4. Add remaining water and shake
vigorously Bottle then contains 100 ml of suspension **Note: This bottle is oversized to
provide greater shake space for ease in reconstitution.** Each 5 ml contains dicloxacillin sodium monohydrate equivalent to 62.5 mg dicloxacillin
*Normal handling may lead to lumps which are not dispersed with continued shaking
©1977 Bristol Laboratories

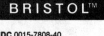

BRISTOL®   NDC 0015-7856-40
                 100 ml BOTTLE

Dynapen®
DICLOXACILLIN
SODIUM FOR ORAL
SUSPENSION
EQUIVALENT TO

62.5 mg per 5 ml

DICLOXACILLIN
when reconstituted according to directions.

CAUTION: Federal law prohibits
dispensing without prescription.

LIFT HERE

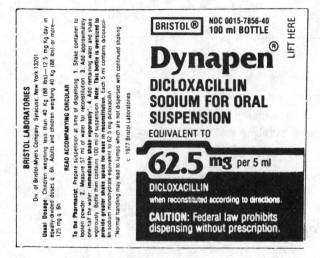

BRISTOL™

NDC 0015-7808-40
100 ml. Bottle

VERSAPEN®
HETACILLIN

FOR ORAL SUSPENSION

EQUIVALENT TO
112.5 mg.
per 5 ml.
AMPICILLIN

when reconstituted
according to directions.

CAUTION: Federal law prohibits
dispensing without prescription.

To the Pharmacist: Prepare suspension at time of dispensing. Add 73 ml. water to the bottle and shake well.
This provides 100 ml. of suspension.

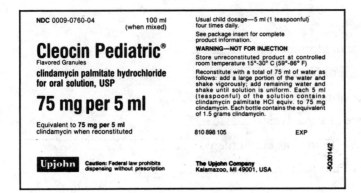

NDC 0009-0760-04   100 ml
(when mixed)

Cleocin Pediatric®
Flavored Granules

clindamycin palmitate hydrochloride
for oral solution, USP

75 mg per 5 ml

Equivalent to 75 mg per 5 ml
clindamycin when reconstituted

Upjohn   Caution: Federal law prohibits
dispensing without prescription

Usual child dosage—5 ml (1 teaspoonful)
four times daily.

See package insert for complete
product information.

WARNING—NOT FOR INJECTION

Store unreconstituted product at controlled
room temperature 15°-30° C (59°-86° F)

Reconstitute with a total of 75 ml of water as
follows: add a large portion of the water and
shake vigorously; add remaining water and
shake until solution is uniform. Each 5 ml
(teaspoonful) of the solution contains
clindamycin palmitate HCl equiv. to 75 mg
clindamycin. Each bottle contains the equivalent
of 1.5 grams clindamycin.

810 898 105   EXP

The Upjohn Company
Kalamazoo, MI 49001, USA

-5Q3014/2

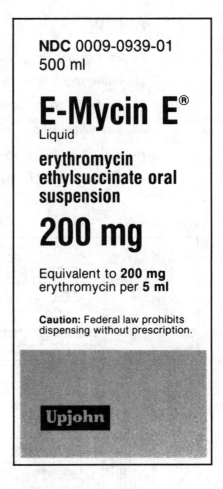

NDC 0009-0939-01
500 ml

E-Mycin E®
Liquid

erythromycin
ethylsuccinate oral
suspension

200 mg

Equivalent to 200 mg
erythromycin per 5 ml

Caution: Federal law prohibits
dispensing without prescription.

Upjohn

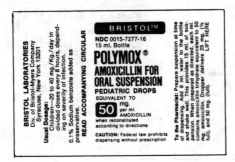

PART III

DIRECTIONS Use the labels provided to calculate the following IM dosages. Calculate to hundredths.

18. Prepare a 20 mg dosage of meperidine. _____

19. A dosage of morphine 10 mg has been ordered. _____

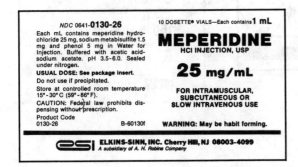

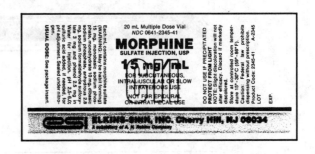

PART IV

20. Prepare a 0.1 mg dosage of atropine. _____

21. Draw up a 100 mg dosage of clindamycin. _____

22. Prepare a 40 mg dosage of meperidine. _____

23. Draw up a 70 mg dosage of kanamycin. _____

24. A dosage of Garamycin® 15 mg has been ordered. _____

25. Prepare a 6 mg dosage of morphine. _____

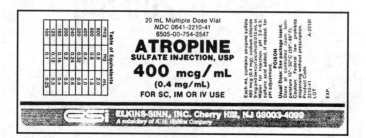

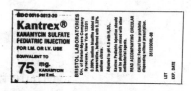

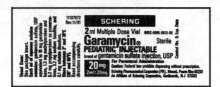

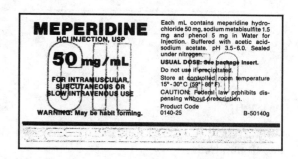

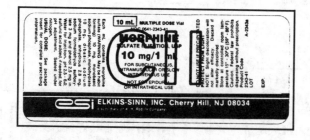

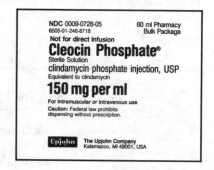

ANSWERS

1. 7.5 mL **2.** 10 mL **3.** 1.5 mL **4.** suspension; mix thoroughly, administer promptly **5.** 11.3 mL **6.** 10 mL **7.** 2.5 mL
8. 0.6 mL **9.** 118 mL of water **10.** 250 mg/5 mL **11.** 6 mL **12.** 10 mL **13.** 6.7 mL **14.** 10 mL **15.** 10 mL **16.** 7.5 mL
17. 1.2 mL **18.** 0.8 mL **19.** 0.67 mL **20.** 0.25 mL **21.** 0.67 mL **22.** 0.8 mL **23.** 1.87 mL **24.** 1.5 mL **25.** 0.6 mL

21
Pediatric Intravenous Medications

OBJECTIVES
The student will
1. list the responsibilities of preparing and administering continuous IV medications
2. list the steps in preparing and administering IV medications on an intermittent basis via Buretrol, Soluset, or Volutrol
3. list the signs and symptoms of IV infiltration and inflammation in an infant or child
4. calculate flow rates for administration of IV medications using the formula or division factor method
5. explain why a flush is included in IV drug administration

INTRODUCTION
Pediatric IV medication administration involves a challenge and a responsibility that is multi-faceted. Infants and children, particularly under the age of four, are incompletely developed physiologically and drug tolerance is a major concern. Infants and acutely ill children can tolerate only a narrow range of hydration and fluid balance making IV drugs, which are diluted for administration, a critical and exact skill.

The fragility of infants' and childrens' veins and the irritating nature of many drugs mandates **careful site inspection for signs of infiltration and inflammation. This should be done immediately before, during and after completion of each medication administration.** Signs of inflammation would include redness, heat, swelling and tenderness. Signs of infiltration include swelling, coldness, pain, and lack of blood return. Either complication necessitates the discontinuing of the IV and a restart at a new site. Close observation of the child's on-going status and communication among nurse, pharmacist and physician is a vital aspect of pediatric IV medication administration.

• METHODS OF IV MEDICATION ADMINISTRATION •

Intravenous medications may be administered **continuously**, for example aminophylline; or on an **intermittent** basis involving several dosages in a 24 hour period, for example antibiotics. When ordered on a **continuous** basis medications are usually added to an IV solution bag, and infused through a primary infusion line. Adding the drug to the IV bag may be an R.N. or hospital pharmacy responsibility, but in any event it is not a complicated procedure. The steps for adding the drug to the solution are as follows:

STEP 1. Locate the type and volume of IV solution ordered.

STEP 2. Measure the dosage of drug to be added.

STEP 3. Use strict aspectic technique to add the drug to the solution bag.

STEP **4.** Label the IV solution bag with the name and dosage of the drug added.

STEP **5.** Add your initials with the time and date you added the drug.

Children receiving IV medications on an **intermittent** basis may or may not have a primary IV running. If a primary line exists, the medication may be administered IVPB (IV piggyback) via a secondary line. If no continuous IV is infusing an indwelling infusion adapter such as the heparin lock (heplock) is frequently used for administration. Medications administered intermittently may be prepared by the pharmacy in small volume infusion bags. These would require only that the label be checked carefully, and that the solution and drug be administered at the correct time and rate.

Intermittent medication dosages are frequently prepared by registered nurses. A special IV set, such as the one shown in figure 79, may be used for the medication preparation. These sets are usually referred to by their trade names, and may be called Buretrols®, Solusets®, or Volutrols® depending on which type is being used. They are **all microdrip sets calibrated to deliver 60 gtt/mL**. The total capacity is between 100 to 150 mL calibrated in 1 mL increments, so that exact measurement of small volumes is possible.

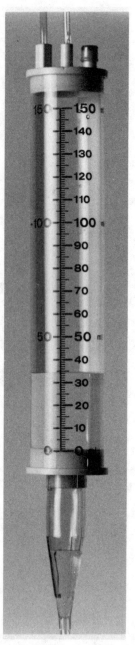

Regardless of the method of intermittent medication administration (IVPB, heplock, or Buretrol) all are followed by a flush to make sure the medication has cleared the IV tubing and the total dosage has been administered. Because hydration is a major concern in pediatrics the flush volume is added to the medication volume for flow rate calculations. For example, a drug may be diluted in 15 mL of solution and followed by a 15 mL flush. The total volume of medication plus flush is 30 mL, and it is this volume which will be used to calculate the flow rate for administration. The solution used for the flush is provided by the primary IV solution, or in the absence of a primary IV, by a solution bag maintained specifically for dilution of medications and flushes. A 15 mL flush is standard for peripheral lines, and 20 mL for central lines. The sequencing of medication and flush administration covered in the next section for Buretrol/Soluset use is also representative of the procedure which would be followed for IVPB and heplock administrations.

• MEDICATION ADMINISTRATION VIA BURETROL •

When a Buretrol is used for medication administration the entire preparation is done by registered nurses. Electronic controllers and pumps are used extensively to regulate and administer intermittent IV medications. When they are used the alarm will sound each time the Buretrol empties to signal when each successive step is necessary. For example it will alarm when the medication has infused and the flush must be started, and again when the flush is completed.

Let's look at some sample orders and go step-by-step through one procedure which may be used.

Figure 79

EXAMPLE 1   Infuse ampicillin 250 mg in 15 mL D5 ½NS over 30 minutes. Follow with 15 mL D5 ½NS flush.

STEP **1.** Read the ampicillin label and determine what volume the 250 mg dosage is contained in. This is 1 mL.

STEP **2.** Determine the flow rate necessary to deliver the medication plus the flush in the 30 minute time period ordered. Either the Formula or the Division Factor method may be used for flow rate calculation.

FORMULA METHOD

$$\text{Flow Rate} = \frac{\text{Total Volume} \times \text{Set Calibration}}{\text{Time in Minutes}}$$

$$\frac{15 \text{ mL (medication)} + 15 \text{ mL (flush)} \times 60 \text{ (gtt/mL)}}{30 \text{ min}}$$

$$\frac{\cancel{30} \times 60}{\cancel{30}} = \textbf{60 gtt/min}$$

DIVISION FACTOR METHOD

$$\text{Flow Rate} = \text{mL/hr} \div \text{Division Factor}$$

To use this method you must express the volume in mL/hr (mL/60 min) equivalents. Use ratio and proportion to determine this.

$$30 \text{ mL} : 30 \text{ min} = X \text{ mL} : 60 \text{ min}$$
$$= 60 \text{ mL in } 60 \text{ min}$$

A 60 gtt/mL set has a division factor of 1 (60 ÷ 60).

$$60 \text{ (mL/hr)} \div 1 \text{ (division factor)} = \textbf{60 gtt/min}$$

The flow rate in gtt/min is the same as the volume in mL/hr for sets calibrated at 60 gtt/mL.

STEP 3. Run a total of 14 mL D5 ½NS into the Buretrol, then add the 1 mL containing the dosage of ampicillin 250 mg. This gives the ordered dilution volume of 15 mL. Roll the Buretrol between your hands to mix the drug thoroughly with the solution.

STEP 4. Adjust the flow rate to deliver 60 gtt/min (60 mL/hr).

STEP 5. Label the Buretrol to identify the drug and dosage added. Attach a label which states "medication infusing". This makes it possible for others to know the status of the administration if you are not present when the controller alarms.

STEP 6. When the medication has infused add the 15 mL D5 ½NS flush. Remove the "medication infusing" label and attach a "flush infusing" label. Continue to infuse at 60 gtt/min until the Buretrol empties for the second time.

STEP 7. When the flush has been completed restart the primary IV, or disconnect from the heplock. Remove the "flush infusing" label.

EXAMPLE 2 An antibiotic dosage of 50 mg has been ordered diluted in 10 mL of D5W to infuse over 20 min. A 15 mL flush of D5W is to follow.

STEP 1. Read the medication label to determine what volume contains 50 mg. You determine that 50 mg is contained in 2 mL.

STEP 2. Determine the flow rate.

Formula Method

$$\frac{10 \text{ mL} + 15 \text{ mL} \times 60 \text{ gtt/mL}}{20 \text{ min}}$$

$$\frac{25 \times 60}{20} = \textbf{75 gtt/min}$$

Division Factor Method 25 mL : 20 min = 75 mL : 60 min

$$= \textbf{75 gtt/min}$$

STEP 3. Run 8 mL of D5W into the Buretrol and add the 2 mL containing 50 mg of drug. Roll between hands to mix.

STEP 4. Set the Buretrol at a rate of 75 gtt/min.

STEP 5. Label the Buretrol with drug name and dosage, and "medication infusing" label.

STEP 6. When the medication has cleared the Buretrol add the 15 mL of D5W flush. Continue to run at 75 gtt/min. Remove the "medication infusing" label and replace with a "flush infusing" label.

STEP 7. When the Buretrol empties for the second time restart the primary IV, or disconnect from the heplock. Remove the "flush infusing" label.

EXAMPLE 3 An antibiotic dosage of 125 mg in 1 mL is to be diluted in 20 mL D5 ¼NS and infused over 30 min. A flush of 15 mL D5 ¼NS is to follow.

Determine the flow rate

Formula Method

$$\frac{20 \text{ mL} + 15 \text{ mL} \times 60 \text{ gtt/mL}}{30 \text{ min}} = \textbf{70 gtt/min}$$

$$\frac{35 \times 60}{30} = \textbf{70 gtt/min}$$

Division Factor Method 35 mL : 30 min = 70 mL : 60 min

$$= \textbf{70 gtt/min}$$

125 mg has a volume of 1 mL. Add 19 mL of D5 ¼NS to the Buretrol, add the 1 mL of medication and mix.

Set the flow rate at 70 gtt/min. Label the Buretrol with the drug and dosage, and attach a "medication infusing" label. When the medication has infused start the 15 mL flush. Remove the "medication infusing" label, and add the "flush infusing" label. When the flush has completed restart the IV or disconnect the heplock. Remove the "flush infusing" label.

PROBLEM

Determine the volume of solution which must be added to the Buretrol to mix the following IV drugs. Then calculate the flow rate for each administration.

1. An IV medication of 75 mg in 3 mL is ordered diluted to 55 mL to infuse over 45 min. A 15 mL flush is to follow. _____ _____

2. A dosage of 100 mg in 2 mL is diluted to 30 mL D5W to infuse in 20 min. A 15 mL flush is to follow. _____ _____

3. The volume of a 10 mg dosage of medication is 1 cc. Dilute to 15 mL and administer over 30 min, with a flush of 15 mL to follow. _____
_____

4. A dosage of 15 mg with a volume of 3 mL is to be diluted to 25 mL and administered in 20 min. A 15 mL flush is to follow. _____ _____

5. A medication of 1 g in 4 mL is to be diluted to 30 mL to infuse over 60 min. A 15 mL flush is to follow. _____ _____

ANSWERS 1. dilute in 52 mL; infuse at 93 gtt/min **2.** dilute in 28 mL; infuse at 135 gtt/min **3.** dilute in 14 mL; infuse at 60 gtt/min **4.** dilute in 22 mL; infuse at 120 gtt/min **5.** dilute in 26 mL; infuse at 45 gtt/min

• IV MEDICATION GUIDELINES/PROTOCOLS •

The variety and complexity of IV drugs being administered on an intermittent basis has prompted many hospitals to develop pediatric administration Guidelines or Protocols for those medications most commonly ordered. These Guidelines represent a compilation of pharmaceutical company recommendations for each drug's use, and include information on dilution, infusion time, maximum concentration, maximum infusion rate, and compatibility with other IV drugs and solutions.

While it is beyond the scope of this text to deal with the details and use of such Guidelines, it is timely to point out that administering IV medications to infants and children will not always be as uncomplicated as the previous routine medication administrations might lead you to believe. We have already mentioned that fluid balance in children is a continuing concern, and on many occasions IV medications may have to be administered at maximum concentration with as small a volume of diluent as possible, in order not to overhydrate a child. Similiary an assessment must be made on the suitability of the flow rate calculated for each child. For example a calculated rate of 100 gtt/min for a child 2 years old is too high a rate to administer. A child's age, size and medical status will often necessitate adjustment of flow rates. Decisions may have to be made on a dose to dose or day to day basis, and will involve the team effort of the nurse, pharmacist and doctor. Your instructor will introduce you to any Guidelines or precautions which are applicable to your specific clinical experience.

This concludes the chapter on administration of IV drugs to infants and children. The important points to remember from this chapter are:

■ intravenous sites must be checked for inflammation and infiltration immediately before, during and following each medication administration

■ IV medications are diluted for administration

■ a flush is used following medication administration to make sure the medication has cleared the tubing and the total dosage has been administered

■ a 15 mL flush is used for peripheral lines and a 20 mL flush for central lines

■ the flow rate for IV medication administration is calculated for the total volume of medication including the flush

■ pediatric IV administration requires constant assessment and adjustment based on a child's age, size, and medical condition

SUMMARY SELF TEST
Pediatric Intravenous Medications

DIRECTIONS Determine the volume of solution which must be added to the Buretrol to mix the following IV drugs. Then calculate the flow rate for each administration.

1. An IV antibiotic of 750 mg in 3 mL has been ordered diluted to a total of 25 mL D5W to infuse over 40 minutes. A flush of 15 mL is to follow. _____

_____

2. A dosage of 500,000 u of a penicillin preparation with a volume of 4 mL has been ordered diluted to 50 mL D5 ½NS to infuse in 60 min. A 15 mL flush has been ordered. _____ _____

3. A dosage of 1.5 g/2 mL of an antibiotic is to be diluted to a total of 40 mL D5W and administered over 40 min. A 15 mL flush has been ordered.

_____ _____

4. An antibiotic dosage of 200 mg in 4 mL is to be diluted in 50 mL and adminis- tered over 60 min. A 20 mL flush has been ordered. _____

_____

5. A dosage of 20 mg in 2 mL has been ordered diluted to 30 mL, to be infused over 30 min. A flush of 15 mL has been ordered. _____

_____

6. A dosage of 25 mg in 5 mL has been ordered diluted to 40 mL and administered in 40 min. A 15 mL flush is to follow. _____ _____

7. A 10 mg in 2 mL dosage has been ordered diluted to 20 mL to infuse over 20 min. A routine 15 mL flush is to follow. _____ _____

8. A dosage of 1000 u has been added to 250 mL of D5W to infuse over 5 hours. What is the flow rate? _____

9. A medication dosage of 800 mg in 4 mL is to be diluted to 60 mL and infused over 60 min. A 15 mL flush is to follow. _____ _____

10. A dosage of 0.5 g in 2 mL is to be diluted to 40 mL and run in 30 min. A 15 mL flush is ordered. _____ _____

11. A medication of 1000 mg in 1 mL is to be diluted to 15 mL and administered over 20 min. A 15 mL flush is ordered. _____ _____

12. A dosage of 40 mg in 4 mL is to be diluted to 50 mL and administered in 90 min. A 20 mL flush is ordered. _____ _____

13. A 2 g in 5 mL dosage has been ordered diluted to a total of 90 mL and administered in 45 min. A 15 mL flush is ordered. _____ _____

14. An 80 mg dosage with a volume of 2 mL is to be diluted to 80 mL and administered in 60 min. A 15 mL flush is to follow. _____ _____

15. A 60 mg dosage with a volume of 4 mL is ordered diluted to 30 mL and run over 20 min. A 15 mL flush is to follow. _____ _____

16. A 5 mg per 2 mL dosage is to be diluted to 10 mL and administered in 10 min. A 15 mL flush follows. _____ _____

17. The dosage ordered is 0.75 g in 3 mL to be diluted to 30 mL. Run in over 30 min with a 15 mL flush. _____ _____

18. A medication of 100 mg in 2 mL is ordered diluted to 20 mL and run in 15 min with a 15 mL flush to follow. _____ _____

19. The dosage ordered is 100 mg in 1 mL to be diluted to 50 mL. Run in over 45 min. Follow with a 15 mL flush. _____ _____

20. A 30 mg dosage in 1 mL has been ordered diluted to 10 mL to infuse in 10 min. A 15 mL flush is ordered. _____ _____

21. A dosage of 250 mg in 5 mL has been ordered diluted to 40 mL and infused in 60 min. A 15 mL flush follows. _____ _____

22. A dosage of 4 mg in 4 mL has been ordered diluted to 30 mL and infused over 40 min. A 15 mL flush is to follow. _____ _____

23. A 15 mg per 3 mL dosage has been ordered diluted to 40 mL and infused over 30 min, with a 15 mL flush to follow. _____ _____

24. A 1.25 g dosage in 5 mL has been ordered diluted to 60 mL and infused over 90 min. A 20 mL flush is to follow. _____ _____

25. A dosage of 450 mg in 3 mL is to be diluted to 30 mL to infuse over 40 min, with a 15 mL flush to follow.

ANSWERS

1. 22 mL, 60 gtt/min   **2.** 46 mL, 65 gtt/min   **3.** 38 mL, 83 gtt/min   **4.** 46 mL, 70 gtt/min   **5.** 28 mL, 90 gtt/min   **6.** 35 mL, 83 gtt/min   **7.** 18 mL, 105 gtt/min   **8.** 50 gtt/min   **9.** 56 mL, 75 gtt/min   **10.** 38 mL, 110 gtt/min   **11.** 14 mL, 90 gtt/min   **12.** 46 mL, 47 gtt/min   **13.** 85 mL, 140 gtt/min   **14.** 78 mL, 95 gtt/min   **15.** 26 mL, 135 gtt/min   **16.** 8 mL, 150 gtt/min   **17.** 27 mL, 90 gtt/min   **18.** 18 mL, 140 gtt/min   **19.** 49 mL, 87 gtt/min   **20.** 9 mL, 150 gtt/min   **21.** 35 mL, 65 gtt/min   **22.** 26 mL, 68 gtt/min   **23.** 37 mL, 110 gtt/min   **24.** 55 mL, 53 gtt/min   **25.** 27 mL, 68 gtt/min

SECTION

SEVEN

Intravenous Medication Calculations

22
IV Flow Rate Calculation

OBJECTIVES
The student will
1. identify calibrations in gtt/mL on IV administration sets
2. calculate flow rates by the formula method
3. calculate flow rates by the division factor method
4. explain the differences in function between electronic controllers and pumps

INTRODUCTION
Intravenous fluids are most frequently ordered on the basis of **mL/hr** to be administered, for example 3000 mL/24 hr, 1000 mL/6 hr, or 125 mL/hr. Smaller volumes, usually containing IV medications, may be ordered in **mL/min**, for example 50 mL/20 min, or 10 mL/5 min. **The volume ordered is administered by adjusting the rate at which the IV runs, or infuses, which is counted in drops per minute (gtt/min).** Most flow rate calculations involve changing mL/hr or mL/min ordered into gtt/min.

Intravenous tubings contain a drip chamber where the drops can be counted. A roller clamp located below the drip chamber is used to adjust the flow to the desired number of gtt/min. The size of the drops is regulated by the size of the IV tubing, but unfortunately all tubings (and drops) are not the same size. **IV tubings are calibrated in gtt/mL**, and this calibration is needed to calculate flow rates.

• IV TUBING CALIBRATION •

Each hospital uses at least two sizes of IV administration tubings. The first is a **standard or macrodrip set**, for use in routine adult IV administrations. The second is called a **mini or microdrip set** and is used when more exact measurements are needed, such as in intensive care and pediatric units, where they are routinely used. Depending on the manufacturer and type of tubing used **it will require 10, 15, or 20 gtt to equal 1 mL in standard macrodrip sets, and 60 gtts to equal 1 mL in mini or microdrip sets**. The calibration, in gtt/mL, is clearly printed on each IV package.

PROBLEM

Refer to the IV tubing packages in figure 80 and identify the calibration in gtt/mL of each.

1. _____

2. _____

3. _____

4. _____

5. _____

1

code 890-02
**60" (152 cm)
I.V. Set**
20 ga x 1½" (3.8 cm) needle
screw clamp
20 Drops=1 ml (approx.)

Cutter

2

TRAVENOL

**minidrip
(approx. 60 drops/ml)**

3

Twin-Site® Venoset®
with CAIR™ Clamp

ABBOTT

No. 8957

15 drops/ml.

100 inch I.V. Set (254 cm.), with CAIR* (constant accurate infusion rate) clamp,
drip chamber providing approximately 15 drops per ml., bacterial retentive air filter,
and two Y injection sites 6 and 39 inches (15 and 99 cm.) from male adapter.
Dimensions are nominal.

*Precision roller clamp mfd. for Abbott by Adelberg R&D Laboratories. U.S. Pat. No. 3,685,787; Canadian Pat. No. 926,371.

4

adapter and remove protector. Attach needle. Open
FLO-TROL clamp. Hold needle upright, fill set and expel
air bubbles. DO NOT ALLOW AIR TO BE TRAPPED IN
SET. Close FLO-TROL clamp and perform venepuncture.
Squeeze and release FLASHBALL site. Blood flashes
back into adapter if needle is in vein. Open FLO-TROL
clamp and regulate flow. (10 drops approx. 1 ml)

FOR SUPPLEMENTARY MEDICATION: Inject supplementary medication with a 20 to 22 gauge needle through
targets on FLASHBALL site or through medication injection
site on solution container. Excessive injection pressure
could cause separation of needle adapter or IV tubing from
FLASHBALL site. DO NOT INJECT SUPPLEMENTARY
MEDICATION INTO THIS SET WHEN DILUTION OF MED-
ICATION IS NECESSARY.

TRAVENOL LABORATORIES, INC.
Deerfield, Illinois 60015, U.S.A.

5

Soluset®
150 x 60
with CAIR® Clamp
Precision Volume I.V. Set

**No. 1882
60 drops/ml.**

Figure 80

• FORMULA METHOD OF FLOW RATE CALCULATION •

When the doctor orders an IV to be infused at a specific mL/hr volume, you will need three pieces of information in order to calculate the flow rate in gtt/min. These are the **total volume to be infused in mL, the calibration of the tubing being used** (which you just learned to locate), **and the time (in minutes) ordered for the infusion**. This information is used in the following formula.

FORMULA

$$\text{Flow Rate} = \frac{\text{Volume} \times \text{Calibration}}{\text{Time (min)}}$$

EXAMPLE 1   The doctor orders an IV to infuse at 125 mL/hr. Calculate the flow rate using a set calibrated at 10 gtt/mL.

Start by converting 1 hour to 60 minutes

$$\frac{125 \text{ (mL)} \times 10 \text{ (gtt/mL)}}{60 \text{ (min)}}$$

$$\frac{125 \times 10}{60} = 20.8 = \textbf{21 gtt/min}$$

Flow rates are routinely rounded off, and answers within 1 gtt/min are considered correct. This IV would be regulated at 21 gtt/min.

EXAMPLE 2   Administer an IV of 100 mL in 40 min using a set calibrated at 15 gtt/mL.

$$\frac{100 \times 15}{40} = 37.5 = \textbf{38 gtt/min}$$

EXAMPLE 3   15 mL of an IV medication is ordered to infuse in 30 min. The set calibration is 60 gtt/mL.

$$\frac{15 \times 60}{30} = \textbf{30 gtt/min}$$

PROBLEM

Calculate the flow rate in gtt/min for the following IV administrations.

1. Administer an IV at 110 mL/hr using a set calibrated at 20 gtt/mL.

   _____

2. An IV is ordered to run at 20 mL/hr using a microdrip set calibrated at 60 gtt/mL.

   _____

3. An IV medication with a volume of 20 mL is to be administered in 20 min using a microdrip set. _____

4. You are to administer 50 mL of an IV antibiotic in 15 min. The set calibration is 10 gtt/mL. _____

5. An IV is ordered to run at 90 mL/hr. The set is calibrated at 15 gtt/mL.

_____

ANSWERS **1.** 37 gtt/min   **2.** 20 gtt/min   **3.** 60 gtt/min   **4.** 33 gtt/min   **5.** 23 gtt/min

The formula method is especially useful for calculating the flow rate of small volumes to be administered in less than an hour. Many medications are given IV in small volume dilutions and this formula works very well for determining the flow rate of these.

When an IV order is written specifying volume to be administered in **more** than one hour the formula can still be used. However, in order to keep the numbers you are working with as small and simple as possible it is best to add a preliminary step, and determine how many **mL/hr** the ordered volume will represent.

EXAMPLE 1 Calculate the flow rate for an IV of 1000 mL to run in over 8 hrs with a set calibrated at 20 gtt/mL.

$$1000 \text{ mL/8hr} = 1000 \div 8 = \textbf{125 mL/hr}$$

$$\frac{125 \text{ (mL)} \times 20 \text{ (gtt/mL)}}{60 \text{ (min)}} = 41.6 = \textbf{42 gtt/min}$$

EXAMPLE 2 2500 mL are to run in over 24 hr with a set calibrated at 10 gtt/mL

$$2500 \div 24 = \textbf{104 mL/hr}$$

$$\frac{104 \times 10}{60} = 17.3 = \textbf{17 gtt/min}$$

EXAMPLE 3 An IV of 1200 mL is ordered to run for 16 hours. Calculate the flow rate if the set is calibrated at 15 gtt/mL.

$$1200 \div 16 = \textbf{75 mL/hr}$$

$$\frac{75 \times 15}{60} = 18.7 = \textbf{19 gtt/min}$$

PROBLEM

Calculate the flow rate in gtt/min for the following infusions.

1. A set with a calibration of 15 gtt/mL is used to infuse 2000 mL in 24 hr.

_____

2. Administer 300 mL in 6 hr. Set is calibrated at 60 gtt/mL. _____

3. Infuse 500 mL in 4 hr. The set calibration is 15 gtt/mL. _____

4. 1200 mL are to be infused in 10 hours. Set calibration is 20 gtt/mL.

_____

5. 500 mL has been ordered to infuse in 5 hours. The set calibration is 10 gtt/mL.

_____

• DIVISION FACTOR METHOD OF FLOW RATE CALCULATION •

A second method called **the division factor method** can be used to determine flow rates. It derives from the same formula you just learned, but **it can only be used if the volume to be administered is expressed in mL/hr (mL/60 min)**. Let's start by looking at how the division factor is obtained.

> Order: Administer an IV at 125 mL/hr. Calibration of the set is 10 gtt/mL (remember that the volume must be expressed as mL/60 min).

$$\frac{125 \text{ (mL)} \times \cancel{10}^{1} \text{ (gtt/mL)}}{\cancel{60}_{6} \text{ (min)}} = 20.8 = \textbf{21 gtt/min}$$

Notice that because you are restricting the time to 60 minutes, the set calibration (10) can be divided into 60 to obtain a constant number (6). **This (6) is the division factor. It can be obtained for any IV administration set by dividing 60 by the calibration of the set.**

PROBLEM

Determine the division factor of the following IV sets.

> **1.** 20 gtt/mL   **2.** 15 gtt/mL   **3.** 60 gtt/mL   **4.** 10 gtt/mL

ANSWERS   **1.** 3   **2.** 4   **3.** 1   **4.** 6

Once you know the division factor, the flow rate can be calculated in one step, by dividing the mL/hr to be administered by the division factor.

FORMULA:

> Flow Rate = mL/hr ÷ Division Factor

EXAMPLE 1   Administer an IV at 100 mL/hr using a set calibrated at 10 gtt/mL

- Determine the division factor

  60 ÷ 10 = **6**

- Calculate the flow rate

  100 ÷ 6 = 16.6 = **17 gtt/min**

EXAMPLE 2   Administer an IV at 125 mL/hr using a set calibrated at 15 gtt/mL.

$$60 \div 15 = 4 \quad 125 \div 4 = 31.2 = \textbf{31 gtt/min}$$

EXAMPLE 3   Administer an IV of 50 mL/hr. Set is calibrated at 60 gtt/mL.

$$60 \div 60 = 1 \quad 50 \div 1 = \textbf{50 gtt/min}$$

Notice that when a microdrip set calibrated at 60 gtt/mL is used, the division factor is 1. Therefore **the flow rate in gtt/min is the same as the volume in mL/hr for microdrip sets**.

EXAMPLE 4   Administer an IV of 80 mL/hr. Set is calibrated at 60 gtt/mL.

$$80 \div 1 = \textbf{80 gtt/min}$$

PROBLEM

Calculate the flow rates for the following IV infusions using the division factor method.

1. Administer 110 mL/hr via a set calibrated at 20 gtt/mL. _____

2. Set is calibrated at 15 gtt/mL. Administer 130 mL/hr. _____

3. Infuse 150 mL in 1 hour. Set calibration is 10 gtt/mL. _____

4. A set calibrated at 60 gtt/mL is used to administer 45 mL/hr. _____

5. Infusion is ordered at the rate of 75 mL/hr with a set calibrated at 15 gtt/mL.

_____

ANSWERS   **1.** 37 gtt/min   **2.** 33 gtt/min   **3.** 25 gtt/min   **4.** 45 gtt/min   **5.** 19 gtt/min

---

The division factor method can be used to calculate the flow rate of any volume that can be expressed in mL/hr. Larger volumes can be divided and expressed in mL/hr, and smaller volumes can be multiplied and expressed in mL/hr.

EXAMPLE 1   2400 mL/24 hr = 2400 $\div$ 24 = 100 mL/hr

EXAMPLE 2   1800 mL/8 hr = 1800 $\div$ 8 = 225 mL/hr

EXAMPLE 3   10 mL/30 min = 10 $\times$ 2 (2 $\times$ 30 min) = 20 mL/hr

EXAMPLE 4   15 mL/20 min = 15 $\times$ 3 (3 $\times$ 20 min) = 45 mL/hr

Once converted to mL/hr equivalents, these administrations can be calculated using the division factor method.

PROBLEM

Calculate the following IV flow rates using the division factor method.

1. An IV of 2000 mL is to infuse in 10 hours using a set calibrated at 20 gtt/mL.

_____

2. An IV antibiotic in 20 mL of solution is to run over 20 minutes with a microdrip.

_____

3. 3000 mL is to infuse IV in the next 24 hours using a 15 gtt/mL set.

_____

4. An IV medication diluted in 30 mL is to infuse in 40 min using a microdrip set.

_____

5. An IV of 100 mL is to run in 30 minutes with a set calibrated at 20 gtt/mL.

_____

ANSWERS   **1.** 67 gtt/min   **2.** 60 gtt/min   **3.** 31 gtt/min   **4.** 45 gtt/min   **5.** 67 gtt/min

• MONITORING IV FLOW RATES •

Uncomplicated IV's are usually administered by straight gravity flow, as illustrated in figure 81.

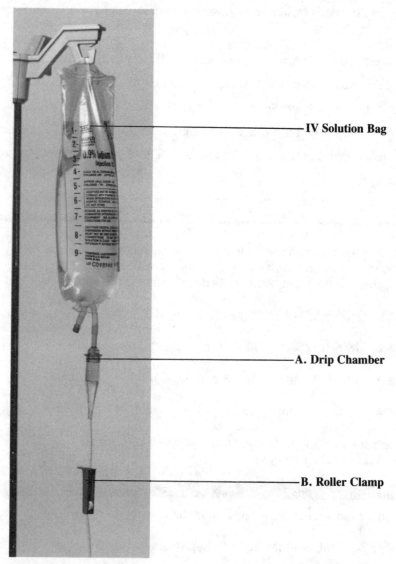

Figure 81

The flow rate is regulated by counting the number of drops falling in the drip chamber (A). The standard procedure for doing this is to actually count the drops for 15 or 30 seconds, and use the roller clamp (B) to adjust the flow rate to the desired gtt/min. For example, if the required rate is 40 gtt/min you would adjust the flow rate to 10 gtt in 15 seconds or 20 gtt in 30 seconds.

PROBLEM

1. The 15 second count of an IV flow rate is 7 gtt. A 29 gtt/min rate is required. Is this rate correct? _____

2. You are to regulate a newly started IV to deliver 67 gtt/min. Using the 15 second count, how would you set the flow rate? _____

3. An IV is to run at 48 gtt/min. What must the drop rate be for 15 seconds?

   _____

ANSWERS **1.** yes   **2.** 16–17 gtt/15 sec   **3.** 12 gtt/15 sec

---

The flow rate changes slightly each time the patient moves, is repositioned, etc., due to pressure changes in the vein and or tubing. For this reason flow rates are routinely checked at least once an hour.

In the majority of hospitals the IV solution bag is labeled with start, finish and progress times to provide a visual reference of the status of the IV. For example the 1000 mL infusion in figure 82 was started at 9 a.m. to run 8 hours (till 5 p.m.). The hourly increments between start and finish are labeled so that, at any time, staff members can check to see that the IV is infusing on schedule.

IV's occasionally infuse ahead of or behind schedule. When this occurs, the common procedure is to recalculate the flow rate using the volume and time remaining, and adjust the rate accordingly. For IV's running behind schedule this also requires an assessment of the patient's ability to tolerate an increased flow rate. If there is any question at all, notify the doctor first.

EXAMPLE 1   An IV of 1000 mL was ordered to infuse over 10 hours at a rate of 25 gtt/min. The set calibration is 15 gtt/mL. After 5 hours you notice that 650 mL have infused instead of the 500 mL ordered. Recalculate the flow rate for the remaining solution.

Time remaining = 5 hours

Volume remaining = 350 mL

350 mL ÷ 5 = 70 mL/hr

Set calibration is 15 gtt/mL

70 ÷ 4 (division factor) = 17.5 = **18 gtt/min**

Slow the rate from 25 gtt/min to 18 gtt/min.

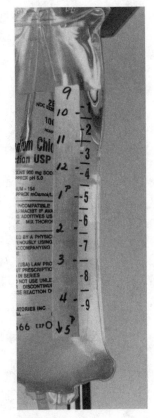

Figure 82

EXAMPLE 2   An IV of 1000 mL was to infuse over 10 hours at 25 gtt/min. After 5 hours you discover that only 300 mL have infused. Recalculate the flow rate using a set calibrated at 15 gtt/mL.

Time remaining = 5 hours

Volume remaining = 700 mL

700 ÷ 5 = 140 mL/hr

140 ÷ 4 = **35 gtt/min**

Increase the rate to 35 gtt/min.

PROBLEM

1. An IV of 500 mL was ordered to infuse in 3 hours using a 15 gtt/mL set. With 1½ hours remaining you discover only 150 mL is left in the bag. At what rate will you need to reset the flow? _____

2. An IV of 1000 mL was scheduled to run in 12 hours. After 4 hours only 220 mL have infused. The set calibration is 20 gtt/mL. Recalculate the rate for the remaining solution. _____

3. An IV of 1000 mL was ordered to infuse in 8 hours. With 3 hours of infusion time left you discover that 600 mL have infused. The set delivers 20 gtt/mL. Recalculate the drip rate and indicate how many drops you will count in 15 seconds to set the new rate. _____ _____

4. An IV of 750 mL was ordered to run over 6 hours with a set calibrated at 10 gtt/mL. After 2 hours you notice that 300 mL have infused. Recalculate the flow rate, and indicate how many drops you will count in 30 seconds to reset the rate.

_____ _____

5. An IV of 800 mL was started at 9 a.m. to infuse in 4 hours. At 10 a.m. 150 mL have infused. The set is calibrated at 15 gtt/mL. Recalculate the flow rate in gtt/min. _____

ANSWERS   1. 25 gtt/min   2. 33 gtt/min   3. 44 gtt/min; 11 gtt/15 sec   4. 19 gtt/min; 9–10 gtt/30 sec
5. 54 gtt/min

• ELECTRONIC IV FLOW RATE REGULATORS •

A variety of electronic IV flow rate regulators are in use in hospitals. These are invaluable assets to IV management because **they can be set to deliver a specific flow rate, and they will alarm if this rate cannot be maintained**. In spite of the variety of models in use, regulators all fit into one of two categories or types: **controllers**, or **pumps** (figure 83). Controllers and pumps look similar physically, but they function differently.

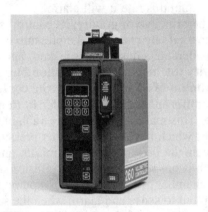
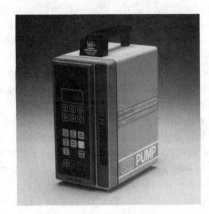

Figure 83

IVAC® Model 260 Controller (left) and Model 560 Volumetric Pump (right). Photos courtesy of IVAC® Corporation.

Controllers work on the same principle of gravity as a regular IV, with the rate of flow being maintained by rapid compression/decompression of the IV tubing by a pincher mechanism inside the controller. Refer to the IVAC® 260 controller model in figure 84.

Notice first that the IV tubing is inserted in the controller at A, where the pincher mechanism is located. A drop sensor, B, is clipped to the tubing's drip chamber. This sensor monitors the flow rate, and causes the controller to adjust and compensate for flow rate changes. The desired flow rate in mL/hr is set on the controller at the flow rate panel, C (some older models may be set in gtt/min). Here is an

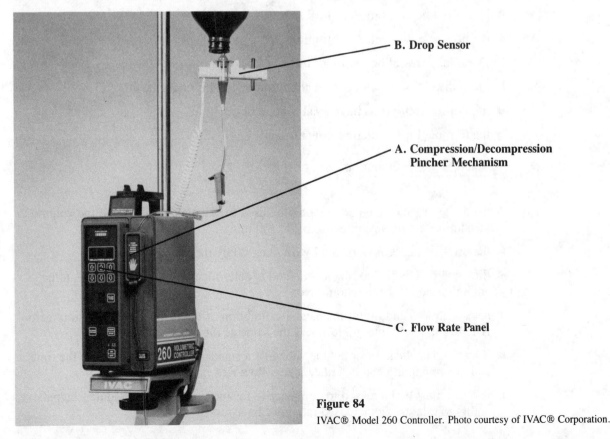

B. Drop Sensor

A. Compression/Decompression Pincher Mechanism

C. Flow Rate Panel

Figure 84

IVAC® Model 260 Controller. Photo courtesy of IVAC® Corporation.

example of how the controller would function. An IV is started, and the controller is set to deliver a rate of 125 mL/hr. Inadvertently the patient rolls on to and partially obstructs the IV tubing. The drip sensor will immediately sense the slowed rate and cause the controller to adjust its compression/decompression cycle to re-establish the pre-set flow rate. If the controller cannot maintain this rate it will alarm.

Remember that a controller works on the principle of gravity; its control is not unlike a roller clamp, in that it adjusts the flow rate by changing the pressure on the IV tubing. The advantage of the controller is that the adjustment is instant, and continuous. **Because controllers work by gravity the height of the solution bag is critical, and must be maintained at a minimum of 36 inches above the controller.**

An electronic "volumetric" pump is different from a controller in that it physically pumps fluids against resistance. This makes it particularly valuable for regulating and infusing fluids through arteries which have a much higher pressure to overcome than infusions into veins. Once again the flow rate is set in mL/hr, and the tubing is positioned through the pump, which is pre-set to deliver the infusion under pressure. A sensor may be used on the drip chamber of the tubing with a pump but its function is not to monitor or adjust the pump but to sense and alarm when the solution bag has emptied. Gravity is not a factor in the use of a pump and the height of the IV solution bag is not a critical factor. As with controllers when the pre-set rate cannot be maintained the pump will alarm.

Use of an electronic regulator does not eliminate the need for visual IV monitoring. The needle site must be checked for inflammation, infiltration, and needle displacement. In addition, the regulators themselves must be monitored to make sure they are functioning properly. Some models also have gauges which visually display resistance pressure to the infusion. By learning to use these correctly, vein resistance and infiltrations can be detected and remedied early.

This concludes the chapter on IV flow rates. The important points to remember from this chapter are:

- IV's are ordered as mL/hr or mL/min to be administered

- the flow rate is counted in gtt/min

- IV tubings are calibrated in gtt/mL

- macrodrip IV sets will have a calibration of 10, 15, or 20 gtt/mL

- mini or microdrip sets have a calibration of 60 gtt/mL

- the formula for calculating flow rates is:

$$\frac{\text{Volume} \times \text{set calibration}}{\text{time (min)}}$$

- the division factor method can only be used to calculate flow rates if the volume to be administered is specified in mL/hr (60 min)

- the division factor is obtained by dividing 60 by the set calibration

- flow rate by the division factor method is determined by dividing the mL to be administered by the division factor

- because micro and minidrips have a calibration of 60 gtt/mL, their division factor is 1, and the flow rate in gtt/min is the same as the mL/hr ordered

- if an IV gets ahead of or behind schedule a standard procedure is to use the time and mL remaining and calculate a new flow rate

- if a rate must be increased to compensate for running behind schedule, the patient's ability to tolerate an increased rate must be assessed

- electronic controllers function by gravity flow and IV's must hang at a minimum of 36″ above the controller

- electronic pumps work by pumping IV fluids under pressure

- frequent IV monitoring by the nurse remains a necessity regardless of the use of electronic regulators

IV Flow Rate Calculation

PART I

1. Refer to the IV administration set packages on page 225 and locate the calibration of the following sets:
   a) Abbott Laboratories Venoset® _____
   b) Cutter IV set   _____
   c) Travenol minidrip   _____

2. Write the formula used for IV flow rate calculations _____

3. Determine the division factor for the following IV sets.
   a) 60 gtt/mL _____
   b) 15 gtt/mL _____
   c) 20 gtt/mL _____
   d) 10 gtt/mL _____

4. How is the flow rate determined in the divison factor method? _____

5. The division factor method can only be used if the volume to be administered is expressed in _____

6. Explain the difference in function between an electronic flow rate controller, and pump. _____

PART II

DIRECTIONS Calculate the flow rate for each of the following IV solutions and medications.

7. D5W 2000 mL has been ordered to run 16 hrs. Set calibration is 10 gtt/mL. _____

8. The order is for 500 mL 0.9% Normal Saline in 8 hrs. The set is calibrated at 15 gtt/mL. _____

9. Administer 150 mL of 5% Sodium Chloride over 3 hrs. A microdrip is used. _____

10. 1500 mL D5W with 40 mEq KCl/L has been ordered to run over 12 hrs. Set calibration is 20 gtt/mL. _____

11. An IV medication of 30 mL is to be administered over 30 min using a 15 gtt/mL set. _____

12. Administer 100 mL 0.9% NaCl in 1 hour using a 15 gtt/mL set. _____

13. Infuse 500 mL intralipids IV in 6 hours. Set calibration is 10 gtt/mL. _____

14. The doctor orders a liter of D5W to infuse over 10 hours. At the end of 8 hours you notice that there is 500 mL left in the bag. What would the new flow rate be if the set calibration is 10 gtt/mL. _____

15. An IV was started at 9 a.m. with orders to infuse 500 mL over 6 hrs. At 12 noon the IV infiltrated with 350 mL left in the bag. At 1 p.m. the IV was restarted. The set calibration is 20 gtt/mL. Calculate the new flow rate to deliver the fluid on time. _____

16. A 50 mL piggyback IV is to infuse over 15 min. The set calibration is 15 gtt/mL. After 5 minutes the IV contains 40 mL. Calculate the flow rate to deliver the volume on time. _____

17. An IV of D5 ¼NS with 20 mEq KCl per liter is ordered to run at 25 mL/hr using a microdrip set. _____

18. Ringers Lactate 800 mL has been ordered to run in over 5 hours. Set calibration is 10 gtt/mL. _____

19. Administer 1500 mL D5 Lactated Ringers solution over 8 hours using a set calibrated at 20 gtt/mL. _____

20. The order is for D5 ½NS 750 mL over 6 hours. Set calibration is 15 gtt/mL.

_____

21. An IV of 1000 mL was ordered to run over 8 hours. After 4 hours only 250 mL have infused. The set calibration is 20 gtt/mL. Recalculate the rate for the remaining solution. _____

22. The order is to infuse 50 mL of a piggyback antibiotic over 1 hour. The set calibration is a microdrip. _____

23. An IV of 500 mL D5W with minocycline 100 mg is to infuse over 6 hours. You will be using a set calibration of 10 gtt/mL. _____

24. Infuse 120 mL gentamicin via IVPB over 1 hour. Set calibration is 10 gtt/mL.

_____

25. Administer 12 mL of an IV medication in 22 min using a microdrip set.

_____

26. A patient is to receive 3000 mL of D5W over 20 hours. Set is calibrated at 20 gtt/mL. _____

27. Infuse 1 liter of D5W over 5 hours using a set calibration of 15 gtt/mL.

_____

28. A hyperalimentation solution of 1180 mL is to infuse over 12 hours using a set calibration of 20 gtt/mL. _____

29. 150 mL of an antibiotic solution is to infuse over 30 minutes. At the end of 20 minutes you discover that 100 mL has infused. The set calibration is 10 gtt/mL. Should the flow rate be adjusted. If so, what is the new rate? _____

30. Two 500 mL units of whole blood are ordered. Both units are to be completed in 5 hours. The set calibration is 20 gtt/mL. _____

31. Infuse 15 mL of IV medication over the next 14 minutes using a 20 gtt/mL set.

_____

32. The patient is to receive 1000 mL 0.9% NaCl in 10 hours using a 20 gtt/mL calibration. _____

33. A minidrip is used to administer 12 mL in 17 minutes. _____

34. Infuse 2750 mL over 20 hours using a 10 gtt/mL set. _____

35. D5W 1800 mL is to infuse in the next 15 hours with a 15 gtt/mL set. _____

36. Infuse 600 mL intralipids IV in 6 hours with a 10 gtt/mL set. _____

37. Administer 22 mL of an IV antibiotic solution in 18 minutes using a minidrip set. _____

38. 1800 mL of D5W with 30 mEq of KCl per liter has been ordered to infuse in 10 hours. Set calibration is 20 gtt/mL. _____

39. Infuse 8 mL in 9 minutes using a minidrip. _____

40. A patient is to receive 4000 mL D5W IV in the next 20 hours. A 20 gtt/mL set is used. _____

ANSWERS

1. a) 15 gtt/mL b) 20 gtt/mL c) 60 gtt/mL   **2.** volume × set calibration ÷ time (min)   **3.** a) 1 b) 4 c) 3 d) 6   **4.** mL/hr ÷ division factor   **5.** mL/hr (mL/60 min)   **6.** controllers function by gravity flow; pumps force fluids under pressure   **7.** 21 gtt/min
8. 16 gtt/min   **9.** 50 gtt/min   **10.** 42 gtt/min   **11.** 15 gtt/min   **12.** 25 gtt/min   **13.** 14 gtt/min   **14.** 42 gtt/min   **15.** 58 gtt/min
16. 60 gtt/min   **17.** 25 gtt/min   **18.** 27 gtt/min   **19.** 63 gtt/min   **20.** 31 gtt/min   **21.** 63 gtt/min   **22.** 50 gtt/min   **23.** 14 gtt/min
24. 20 gtt/min   **25.** 33 gtt/min   **26.** 50 gtt/min   **27.** 50 gtt/min   **28.** 33 gtt/min   **29.** No, rate is correct at 50 gtt/min
30. 67 gtt/min   **31.** 21 gtt/min   **32.** 33 gtt/min   **33.** 42 gtt/min   **34.** 23 gtt/min   **35.** 30 gtt/min   **36.** 17 gtt/min   **37.** 73 gtt/min
38. 60 gtt/min   **39.** 53 gtt/min   **40.** 67 gtt/min

23
Calculating IV Infusion Times

OBJECTIVES
The student will calculate IV infusion times using
1. mL/hr ordered
2. gtt/min and set calibration

INTRODUCTION
The infusion time is the total time necessary for a given volume of solution to infuse intravenously. This time may be within a number of minutes, hours or days depending on the type of solution and the individual patient needs. The total time required for the infusion to be completed is determined by three factors: volume to be infused, drip rate, and set calibration. Once these factors are known the total infusion time can be quickly calculated. It is good planning to have the next solution prepared and ready to hang before the present one is completed. Determining infusion times is also important because laboratory studies are often made before, during, or after specified amounts of IV solutions have infused. It is your responsibility to accurately calculate all IV rates and times.

• BASIC INFUSION TIME FORMULA •

An easy one step formula is used to determine the infusion time. **Always determine first how many mL/hr the patient is receiving, then set up the formula.**

FORMULA

$$\text{Infusion Time} = \frac{\text{total volume to infuse}}{\text{mL/hr being infused}}$$

EXAMPLE 1   Calculate the infusion time for an IV of 500 mL D5W that is infusing at 50 mL/hr.

$$\frac{500 \text{ mL}}{50 \text{ mL/hr}} = 500 \text{ (mL)} \div 50 \text{ (mL/hr)} = \textbf{10 hours}$$

Infusion time = 10 hours

EXAMPLE 2   A doctor orders 1000 mL of D5NS to infuse at 75 mL/hr. Calculate the infusion time.

$$\frac{1000 \text{ mL}}{75 \text{ mL/hr}} = 13.33$$

In this example the 13 represents 13 hours, while .33 represents a fraction of an additional hour. To convert .33 to minutes multiply by 60 (min).

$60 \times .33 = 19.8 =$ **20 min**   Round off the minutes to the nearest whole number

Infusion time = 13 hr 20 min

EXAMPLE 3   A patient has an IV of 1000 mL 5% D5W infusing at 90 mL/hr. How many hours will it take this IV to complete?

$$\frac{1000 \text{ mL}}{90 \text{ mL/hr}} = 11.11$$

$.11 \times 60 \text{ min} = 6.6 \text{ or } 7$

Infusion time = 11 hr 7 min

If the IV was started at 7:30 a.m., at what time will it be completed?

Answer: 6:37 p.m.

PROBLEM

An IV of 900 mL RL is ordered to infuse at a rate of 80 mL/hr. Determine the infusion time.

a) 11 hr 15 min   b) 11 hr 25 min

ANSWER   The correct answer is a), 11 hr 15 min

Remember the 11 represents hours, but the .25 is not minutes, it is a fraction of an additional hour. Convert this to minutes by multiplying 60 by .25

PROBLEM

The doctor orders a volume of 250 mL to be infused at 30 mL per hour. You start the infusion at 12 noon. Calculate the infusion time. When will the IV be completed?

Infusion time _____   Time completed _____

ANSWER   The infusion time is 8 hr 20 min. The IV will be completed at 8:20 p.m.

PROBLEM

A volume of 180 mL of NS is ordered to infuse at 25 mL/hr. Calculate the infusion time.

ANSWER   Infusion time = 7 hr 12 min

• CALCULATING FROM GTT/MIN and SET CALIBRATION •

In some instances the only information you may have is the total volume to infuse, the gtt/min the IV is infusing at, and the set calibration of the tubing. You still use the same infusion time formula but first must convert gtt/min to mL/hr. This is done in a 2 step procedure using ratio and proportion. Here's how.

EXAMPLE 1   Calculate the infusion time for an IV of 1000 mL of D5W running at 25 gtt/min using a set calibrated at 10 gtt/mL.

■ To determine the number of mL/hr the IV is infusing at, first **convert gtt/min to mL/min infusing**

$$10 \text{ gtt} : 1 \text{ mL} = 25 \text{ gtt} : X \text{ mL}$$
$$25 = 10X$$
$$25 \div 10 = X = \textbf{2.5 mL/min}$$

■ **Next, convert mL/min to mL/hr**

$$2.5 \text{ mL/min} \times 60 \text{ (min)} = \textbf{150 mL/hr}$$

■ **Now determine the infusion time using the same basic formula**

$$\frac{1000 \text{ mL}}{150 \text{ (mL/hr)}} = 6.67$$

$$60 \text{ min} \times .67 = 40 \text{ min}$$

Infusion time = 6 hr 40 min

EXAMPLE 2   A patient is to receive 750 mL D5RL at a flow rate of 12 gtt/min using a set calibration of 10 gtt/mL. Calculate the infusion time.

■ **Convert gtt/min to mL/min**

$$10 \text{ gtt} : 1 \text{ mL} = 12 \text{ gtt} : X \text{ mL}$$
$$12 = 10X$$
$$X = \textbf{1.2 mL/min}$$

■ **Convert mL/min to mL/hr**

$$1.2 \text{ mL/min} \times 60 \text{ min} = \textbf{72 mL/hr}$$

■ **Calculate infusion time**

$$\frac{750 \text{ mL}}{72 \text{ mL/hr}} = 10.42$$

$$60 \text{ min} \times .42 = 25 \text{ min}$$

Infusion time = 10 hr 25 min

EXAMPLE 3   Using a microdrip set, determine the infusion time of 100 mL of D5NS
infusing at a rate of 40 gtt/min.

- ■ **Convert gtt/min to mL/min**

$$60 \text{ gtt} : 1 \text{ mL} = 40 \text{ gtt} : X \text{ mL}$$
$$40 = 60X$$
$$X = \textbf{0.67 mL/min}$$

- ■ **Convert mL/min to mL/hr**

$$0.67 \text{ mL/min} \times 60 \text{ min} = \textbf{40 mL/hr}$$

- ■ **Calculate infusion time**

$$\frac{100 \text{ mL}}{40 \text{ mL/hr}} = 2.5$$

$$60 \text{ min} \times .5 = 30 \text{ min}$$

Infusion time = 2 hr 30 min

PROBLEM

1. Calculate the infusion time of an IV that has a volume of 150 mL and is infusing
at 20 gtt/min using a set calibration of 15 gtt/mL. _____

2. The order is to infuse 1100 mL of hyperalimentation solution. The set calibration
is 10 gtt/mL and the flow rate is 10 gtt/min. Calculate the infusion time.

_____

ANSWERS   1. 1 hr 55 min   **2.** 18 hr 20 min

1. Solution:

- ■ $15 \text{ gtt} : 1 \text{ mL} = 20 \text{ gtt} : X \text{ mL}$
$$20 = 15X$$
$$X = \textbf{1.3 mL/min}$$

- ■ $1.3 \text{ mL/min} \times 60 \text{ min} = 78 \text{ mL/hr}$

- ■ $\dfrac{150 \text{ mL}}{78 \text{ mL/hr}} = \textbf{1.92}$

- ■ $.92 \times 60 \text{ min} = \textbf{55 min}$

Infusion time = 1 hr 55 min

2. Solution:

- ■ $10 \text{ gtt} : 1 \text{ mL} = 10 \text{ gtt} : X \text{ mL}$
$$10 = 10X$$
$$X = \textbf{1 mL/min}$$

■ 1 mL/min × 60 min = 60 mL/hr

■ $\dfrac{1100 \text{ mL}}{60 \text{ mL/hr}} = \textbf{18.33}$

■ .33 × 60 min = **20 min**

Infusion time = 18 hr 20 min

PROBLEM

3. Determine the infusion time of 1 liter 5%DW at a flow rate of 33 gtt/min and a set calibration of 15 gtt/mL. _____

4. The doctor asks at what time a patient's infusion will be completed. There is 250 mL left in the IV with a flow rate of 25 gtt/min and set calibration of 10 gtt/mL. The time is now 1 p.m. _____

5. A volume of 100 mL is ordered to infuse at 10 gtt/min. The set calibration of the tubing is 10 gtt/mL. Calculate the infusion time. _____

ANSWERS   **3.** 7 hr 35 min   **4.** 2:40 p.m.   **5.** 1 hr 40 min

The infusion time may vary by several minutes depending on whether you round off to the nearest hundredth, or tenth. Variations of a few minutes are generally not considered significant. If you are having any difficulty with these calculations review all the examples and solutions carefully once again.

• FORMULA METHOD FOR CALCULATING INFUSION TIMES •

For those who prefer working with formulas rather than straight ratio and proportion here is a second way of calculating infusion times. This formula uses the **volume to infuse, the gtt/min, and set calibration**. If the gtt/min or set calibration is not known this formula cannot be used.

FORMULA

$$\text{Total volume to infuse} \div \left(\frac{\text{gtt/min}}{\text{set calibration}} \times 60 \text{ min} \right)$$

Let's begin with a few examples that will illustrate this method.

EXAMPLE 1   There are 250 mL of dextrose in an IV piggyback that is infusing at 33 gtt/min and the set calibration is 10 gtt/mL. Calculate the infusion time.

■ $250 \text{ mL} \div \dfrac{33 \text{ gtt/min}}{10 \text{ gtt/mL}} \times 60$

- 250 mL ÷ 198 mL/hr = 1.26

- .26 × 60 min = 16

- **Infusion time = 1 hr 16 min**

EXAMPLE 2   There are 500 mL of whole blood infusing at 40 gtt/min with a set calibration of 20 gtt/mL. Determine the infusion time.

- $500 \text{ mL} \div \dfrac{40 \text{ gtt/min}}{20 \text{ gtt/mL}} \times 60 \text{ min}$

- 500 mL ÷ 120 mL/hr = 4.17

- .17 × 60 min = 10

- **Infusion time = 4 hr 10 min**

EXAMPLE 3   Infuse 1150 mL of hyperalimentation at 25 gtt/min using a set calibration of 10 gtt/mL. Calculate the infusion time.

- $1150 \text{ mL} \div \dfrac{25 \text{ gtt/min}}{10 \text{ gtt/mL}} \times 60 \text{ min}$

- 1150 mL ÷ 150 mL/hr = 7.67

- .67 × 60 min = 40

- **Infusion time 7 hr 40 min**

PROBLEM

Determine the following infusion times using the formula method.

1. 450 mL D5NS—set calibration 20 gtt/mL—flow rate 25 gtt/min _____

2. 1000 mL D5W—set calibration 10 gtt/mL—flow rate 33 gtt/min _____

3. 150 mL—flow rate 15 gtt/min—set calibration 15 gtt/mL _____

4. 50 mL—flow rate 10 gtt/min—set calibration 15 gtt/mL _____

ANSWERS   **1.** 6 hr   **2.** 5 hr 3 min   **3.** 2 hr 30 min   **4.** 1 hr 15 min

Remember that this formula method will only work when you know the gtt/min and the set calibration of the tubing. After you have worked and practiced with these methods you may select the one which works the best and most consistently for you and then stick with that method.

This concludes the chapter on infusion times. The important points to remember from this chapter are:

- the infusion time is the total time necessary for a given volume of solution to infuse

- there are two methods to determine infusion times:

$$\text{Formula 1: Infusion time} = \frac{\text{total volume to infuse}}{\text{mL/hr being infused}}$$

$$\text{Formula 2: Total volume to infuse} \div \frac{\text{gtt/min} \times 60 \text{ min}}{\text{set calibration}}$$

- the Formula 2 method can only be used when you know the gtt/min and the calibration of the tubing

- in many instances the only information you will have available will be the gtt/min the IV is infusing at and the set calibration of the tubing. In this case either the ratio and proportion method or the formula 2 method can be used

For further practice of infusion times and mastery of these calculations complete the following Summary Self Test. Look carefully at the data provided in each of the questions and ask yourself what information you need before setting up the problem. Sometimes there may be more data than you need to do the problem. The methods previously explained in this chapter take some time and thought to make sense. However, once you've mastered these, calculating infusion times becomes easy.

SUMMARY SELF TEST

Calculating IV Infusion Times

DIRECTIONS　Calculate the following infusion times using any of the methods above.

1. Order: 50 mL D5W with 1 g Kefzol. The flow rate is 50 gtt/min, set calibration is a microdrip.
   Infusion time: _____

2. Infuse 1150 mL hyperalimentation at 80 mL per hour.
   Infusion time: _____

3. There is 280 mL left in the IV bag. The flow rate is 40 gtt/min and the set calibration is 10 gtt/mL.
   Infusion time: _____

4. Order: Infuse 500 mL of whole blood at 30 gtt/min using a set calibration of 20 gtt/mL.
   Infusion time: _____

5. You find 850 mL left in your patient's IV. The time is 10 a.m. The IV is infusing at 25 gtt/min with a set calibration of 10 gtt/mL. At what time will the infusion be completed?
   Infusion time: _____　　**Time completed** _____

6. Infuse 500 mL of Intralipids at 25 mL/hr.
   Infusion time: _____

7. A piggyback has 50 mL of solution infusing at 30 gtt/min. The set calibration is 15 gtt/mL.
   Infusion time: _____

8. There are 520 mL in the IV bag. Set calibration is 15 gtt/mL and the flow rate is 22 gtt/min.
   Infusion time: _____

9. The time is 12 p.m. and there is 900 mL left in the present IV. The flow rate is 50 mL/hr and the set calibration is 10 gtt/min. When will the IV be completed?
   Infusion time: _____　　**Time completed** _____

10. Infuse 150 mL of an antibiotic at 33 gtt/min. Set calibration is 10 gtt/mL.
    Infusion time: _____

11. Order: Infuse 250 mL of packed red blood cells at 20 mL/hr.
    Infusion time: _____

12. The flow rate for 1 liter of D5W is 42 gtt/min. Set calibration is 15 gtt/mL.
    Infusion time: _____

13. Infuse 1 unit of packed cells at a flow rate of 30 gtt/min. One unit contains 250 mL. The set calibration is 20 gtt/mL. Calculate entire infusion time.
    Infusion time: _____

14. Volume to infuse is 100 mL. Flow rate is 42 gtt/min using a microdrip.
    Infusion time: _____

15. At 11 p.m. you notice that 200 mL remains in the IV. The flow rate is 20 gtt/min and the set calibration is 10 gtt/mL. What time can you expect the IV to complete?
    Infusion time: _____ **Time completed** _____

16. A fluid challenge of 350 mL IV is ordered to infuse at 50 gtt/min. Set calibration is 10 gtt/mL.
    Infusion time: _____

17. An infant is to receive 25 mL of solution at 25 gtt/min. The set calibration is 60 gtt/mL.
    Infusion time: _____

18. 425 mL of D5 ½NS is infusing at 15 gtt/min. The set calibration is 10 gtt/mL.
    Infusion time: _____

19. There are 180 mL left in an IV that is infusing at 25 mL/hr. It is 10:30 p.m. What time will it be completed?
    Infusion time: _____ **Time completed** _____

20. At 2 p.m. a nurse starts 500 mL of solution, and regulates the flow rate at 20 gtt/min. The set calibration is 20 gtt/mL. At what time will the infusion be completed?
    Infusion time: _____ **Time completed** _____

21. Order: Infuse 250 mL of NS at 50 gtt/min. Set calibration is 15 gtt/mL.
    Infusion time: _____

22. A physician orders an IV rate to be reduced from 50 gtt/min to 35 gtt/min. There are 525 mL left to infuse. Set calibration is 10 gtt/mL.
    Infusion time: _____

23. A liter of D5 ¼NS with 10 u regular insulin has just been started and is infusing at 22 gtt/min. Set calibration is 20 gtt/mL.
    Infusion time: _____

24. A physician orders 2 liters of 0.9% NS to infuse at 200 mL/hr.
    Infusion time: _____

25. An antibiotic solution of 100 mL is running at 33 gtt/min with a set calibration of 10 gtt/mL.
    Infusion time: _____

ANSWERS

1. 1 hr **2.** 14 hr 23 min **3.** 1 hr 10 min **4.** 5 hr 34 min **5.** 5 hr 40 min; 3:40 p.m. **6.** 20 hr **7.** 25 min **8.** 5 hr 55 min
9. 18 hr; 6 a.m. **10.** 46 min **11.** 12 hr 30 mins **12.** 5 hr 57 min **13.** 2 hr 42 min **14.** 2 hr 23 min **15.** 1 hr 40 min; 12:40 a.m.
16. 1 hr 10 min **17.** 1 hr **18.** 4 hr 43 min **19.** 7 hr 12 min; 5:42 a.m. **20.** 8 hr 20 min; 10:20 p.m. **21.** 1 hr 15 min
22. 2 hr 30 min **23.** 15 hr 9 min **24.** 10 hr **25.** 31 min

24
Calculating Heparin Infusions

OBJECTIVES

The student will calculate
1. hourly heparin dosages
2. heparin flow rates

INTRODUCTION

Heparin is an anticoagulant which is frequently ordered IV to infuse at a specific flow rate per hour, or by a unit dosage per hour. Because of the nature of this drug and its potential side effects it is necessary to carefully monitor the dosage either hourly or daily. Whether you administer heparin via a volumetric pump or by standard IV tubing, determining the dosage and flow rate is your responsibility. The dosage of heparin is expressed in USP units. The requirement for full-dose therapy varies greatly with each patient and is carefully individualized based on body weight and clinical laboratory findings in order to obtain the optimum therapeutic effects. This chapter will teach you how to calculate hourly dosages and flow rates of heparin using the method of ratio and proportion.

• CALCULATING THE HOURLY DOSAGE •

If a heparin order asks that you infuse an IV at a predetermined flow rate the physician has already calculated the dosage per hour of heparin the patient is to receive. However, it still remains a nursing responsibility to calculate the dosage per hour and to assure the safe administration of the drug. Look closely at the following examples.

EXAMPLE 1 An IV of 1000 mL D5W containing 40,000 u heparin has been ordered to infuse at 30 mL/hr. Calculate the dosage of heparin the patient is receiving per hour.

40,000 u : 1000 mL = X u : 30 mL

40,000 × 30 = 1000X

2,000,000 ÷ 1000 = X = **1200 u/hr**

The patient is receiving 1200 u of heparin per hour

The normal heparinizing dosage for adults is 20,000–40,000 u every 24 hr. Is the patient receiving the recommended dosage?

1200 u/hr × 24/hr = **28,800 u/24 hr**. This dosage is within the therapeutic range for adults.

EXAMPLE 2   Order: Add 20,000 u heparin to 1 L D5NS and infuse at 80 mL/hr. Calculate the hourly heparin dosage. Is the dose within the normal recommended range?

$$20,000 \text{ u} : 1000 \text{ mL} = \text{X u} : 80 \text{ mL}$$

$$20,000 \times 80 = 1000\text{X}$$

$$1,600,000 \div 1000 = \text{X} = \textbf{1600 u/hr}$$

1600 u/hr $\times$ 24 hr = **38,400 u/24 hr**. This dose is within the normal therapeutic range.

EXAMPLE 3   An IV of D5W 500 mL with 10,000 u heparin is infusing at 30 mL/hr. Calculate the hourly dosage and determine if the dose is within normal range.

$$10,000 \text{ u} : 500 \text{ mL} = \text{X u} : 30 \text{ mL}$$

$$10,000 \times 30 = 500\text{X}$$

$$300,000 \div 500 = \text{X} = \textbf{600 u/hr}$$

600 u $\times$ 24 = **14,400 u/24 hr**. This is less than the recommended dosage and the physcian should be notified and the order clarified.

PROBLEM

Calculate the following hourly heparin dosages and determine if they are within the recommended heparinizing range.

1. Order: Add 30,000 u heparin to 750 mL D5W and infuse at 25 mL/hr.

   _____

2. A 20,000 u vial of heparin is added to 500 mL D5W and is ordered to infuse at 30 mL/hr. _____

3. One liter of D5NS is started with 60,000 u of heparin IV. Doctors orders are to infuse at 40 mL/hr. _____

4. Order: Add 50,000 u heparin to 1 liter D5W and infuse at 75 mL/hr.

   _____

5. A nurse adds 25,000 u heparin to 500 mL D5W and begins the ordered infusion at 30 mL/hr. _____

6. Order: Add 20,000 u heparin to 1 liter of D5 1/2NS and infuse at 90 mL/hr.

   _____

7. An IV of 500 mL D5W with 40,000 u heparin is started at 25 mL/hr.

   _____

8. A newly written order is for 1 liter of D5NS with 50,000 u heparin to infuse at 25 mL/hr. _____

ANSWERS   1. 1000 u/hr, within normal range   **2.** 1200 u/hr, within normal range   **3.** 2400 u/hr, above normal range   **4.** 3750 u/hr, above normal range   **5.** 1500 u/hr, within normal range   **6.** 1800 u/hr, above normal range   **7.** 2000 u/hr, above normal range   **8.** 1250 u/hr, within normal range

---

• CALCULATING HOURLY DOSAGES FROM SET CALIBRATION AND FLOW RATE •

Heparin dosages may be calculated hourly from set calibration and flow rate information only. This calculation involves several steps. **First the volume in mL/hr being infused is calculated.** Once this is obtained the same ratio and proportion method is used to determine the heparin dosage being given. Let's look at some examples.

EXAMPLE 1   Calculate the hourly heparin dosage a patient is receiving if the solution contains 25,000 u in 1 L D5W. The set calibration is 15 gtt/mL and the IV flow rate is 30 gtt/min.

- **Convert gtt/min to mL/min**

  15 gtt : 1 mL = 30 gtt : X mL
  X = **2 mL/min**

- **Convert mL/min to mL/hr**

  2 mL/min × 60 min = **120 mL/hr**

- **Calculate units per hour**

  25,000 u : 1000 mL = X u : 120 mL
  X = **3000 u/hr**

The patient is receiving 3000 u of heparin per hour.

EXAMPLE 2   A new IV of 1000 mL D5W with 20,000 u of heparin is infusing at 12 gtt/min. The set calibration is 10 gtt/mL. Calculate the hourly dosage of heparin.

- **Convert gtt/min to mL/min**

  10 gtt : 1 mL = 12 gtt : X mL
  X = **1.2 mL/min**

- **Convert mL/min to mL/hr**

  1.2 mL/min × 60 min = **72 mL/hr**

- **Calculate units per hour**

  20,000 u : 1000 mL = X u : 72 mL
  X = **1440 u/hr**

The patient is receiving 1440 u/hr

EXAMPLE 3 The patient has an IV of 25,000 u of heparin in 1 L D5W infusing at 10 gtt/min. Using a set calibration of 15 gtt/mL determine the hourly heparin dosage. Round off to the nearest hundredth.

- **Convert gtt/min to mL/min**

    15 gtt : 1 mL = 10 gtt : X mL
         X = **0.67 mL/min**

- **Convert mL/min to mL/hr**

    0.67 mL/min × 60 min = **40 mL/hr**

- **Calculate units per hour**

    25,000 u : 1000 mL = X u : 40 mL
            X = **1000 u/hr**

The patient is receiving 1000 u/hr

EXAMPLE 4 Calculate the hourly heparin dosage of a patient who has an IV of 1000 mL D5 ¼NS with 60,000 u heparin that is infusing at 30 gtt/min and has a set calibration of 60 gtt/mL.

- **Convert gtt/min to mL/min**

    60 gtt : 1 mL = 30 gtt : X mL
         X = **0.5 mL/min**

- **Convert mL/min to mL/hr**

    0.5 mL/min × 60 min = **30 mL/hr**

- **Calculate units per hour**

    60,000 u : 1000 mL = X u : 30 mL
            X = **1800 u/hr**

PROBLEM

Calculate the dosage of heparin each patient is receiving hourly in the following problems.

1. A liter of D5NS with 40,000 u of heparin is infusing IV at 12 gtt/min. The set calibration is 20 gtt/mL. _____

2. A patient is receiving an IV of 500 mL D5W with 25,000 u heparin which is infusing at 10 gtt/min. The tubing administers 10 gtt/mL. _____

3. Orders are to infuse 1 liter of IV solution containing 10,000 u heparin at 20 gtt/min using a set calibration of 15 gtt/mL. _____

4. Your patient has a new IV of 1 L D5W with 30,000 u of heparin infusing at 8 gtt/min. The set calibration is 15 gtt/mL. _____

5. 500 mL of D5W with 25,000 u of heparin is infusing at 25 gtt/min using a set calibration of 60 gtt/mL. _____

ANSWERS   **1.** 1440 u/hr   **2.** 3000 u/hr   **3.** 800 u/hr   **4.** 960 u/hr   **5.** 1250 u/hr

---

• CALCULATING HEPARIN FLOW RATES •

Heparin is frequently ordered in **units per hour** to be administered. In this situation you must **first calculate how many mL/hr will contain the units ordered, then determine the flow rate necessary to deliver this amount.**

EXAMPLE 1   Order: Infuse 1000 u/hr of heparin IV from a solution of 20,000 u in 500 mL D5W. The administration set is a microdrip. Calculate the flow rate.

■ **Calculate mL/hr to be administered**

$$20,000 \text{ u} : 500 \text{ mL} = 1000 \text{ u} : X \text{ mL}$$
$$500 \times 1000 = 20,000X$$
$$X = \textbf{25 mL/hr}$$

■ **Calculate the flow rate in gtt/min**
The set available is a microdrip

$$25 \text{ mL/hr} \div 1 \text{ (division factor)} = \textbf{25 gtt/min}$$

EXAMPLE 2   The doctor orders heparin 800 u/hr IV. Solution available is 40,000 u in 1000 mL D5W. Set calibration is 15 gtt/mL. Calculate the flow rate.

■ **Calculate mL/hr**

$$40,000 \text{ u} : 1000 \text{ mL} = 800 \text{ u} : X \text{ mL}$$
$$1000 \times 800 = 40,000X$$
$$X = \textbf{20 mL/hr}$$

■ **Calculate the flow rate in gtt/min**

$$20 \text{ mL/hr} \div 4 \text{ (division factor)} = \textbf{5 gtt/min}$$

EXAMPLE 3   Order: Infuse 1200 u/hr of heparin IV. Solution available is 60,000 u in 1 L D5W. Set calibration is 20 gtt/mL.

■ **Calculate mL/hr**

$$60,000 \text{ u} : 1000 \text{ mL} = 1200 \text{ u} : X \text{ mL}$$
$$1000 \times 1200 = 60,000X$$
$$X = 20 \text{ mL/hr}$$

■ **Calculate the flow rate in gtt/min**

20 mL/hr ÷ 3 (division factor) = **6.6 or 7 gtt/min**

PROBLEM

Calculate the flow rates in gtt/min of the following.

1. Administer 1000 u heparin IV every hour. Solution available is 25,000 u in 500 mL of D5W. Set calibration is a microdrip. _____

2. A patient with deep vein thrombosis has orders for heparin 10,000 u every 4 hours IV continuously. Solution available is 50,000 u in 1000 mL D5W. The set calibration is 20 gtt/mL. _____

3. Order: Give 1100 u/hr of heparin IV. Solution 15,000 u in 1 L D5NS. Set calibration is 10 gtt/mL. _____

4. Your newly admitted patient has orders to mix 50,000 u of heparin in 1 L D5W and infuse 2000 u/hr continuously. Set calibration is 15 gtt/mL. _____

5. Administer 1500 u/hr of heparin IV using a solution of 40,000 u in 750 mL D5 ½NS. Set calibration is 60 gtt/mL. _____

ANSWERS **1.** 20 gtt/min **2.** 17 gtt/min **3.** 12 gtt/min **4.** 10 gtt/min **5.** 28 gtt/min

This ends the chapter on IV heparin calculations. The important points to remember are:

■ heparin dosages are highly individualized and may be ordered by flow rate, or units per hour

■ the normal heparinizing dosage for adults is between 20,000–40,000 u every 24 hours

■ hourly heparin dosages may be calculated from the set calibration of the tubing and the flow rate

■ when heparin is ordered in units per hour, first determine the number of mL/hr the patient should receive, then determine the actual flow rate

■ although we have focused only on the administration of heparin in this chapter, it is intended that the information and calculations learned here be applied to other IV medications you will be administering in the future

SUMMARY SELF TEST

Calculating Heparin Infusions

DIRECTIONS Calculate the following heparin dosages and flow rates.

1. The doctor orders a patient to receive 6000 u of heparin every 6 hours continuously IV. The solution available is 25,000 u in 1 L of D5W. The set calibration is 60 gtt/mL. Calculate the correct flow rate. _____

2. A solution of 25,000 u heparin in 1 L D5 ¼NS is infusing at 15 gtt/min. The tubing set delivers 10 gtt/mL. Calculate the hourly heparin dosage. _____

3. A doctor orders a patient to receive 1200 u of heparin every hour IV continuously. The solution is 35,000 u heparin in 1 L D5 ½NS. Calculate the mL/hr the patient will receive. _____

4. There is 20,000 u of heparin in 500 mL D5W infusing at 40 mL per hour. Calculate the hourly unit dosage. _____

5. A newly admitted patient is to receive 1250 u of heparin per hour continuously. The solution available is 1 L D5 ¼NS with 50,000 u heparin. Set calibration is 15 gtt/mL. Calculate the hourly flow rate and gtt/min. _____

6. To help prevent further pulmonary emboli a physician orders 5000 u of heparin IV every 2 hours continuously. The available solution is 40,000 u in 1 L D5RL. Calculate the flow rate if the set calibration is 10 gtt/mL. _____

7. Order: Infuse a solution of 25,000 u heparin in 1 L D5W over 24 hours. Calculate the hourly unit dosage, then the flow rate using a set calibration of 10 gtt/mL. _____

8. Calculate the hourly unit dosage of heparin and determine if it is within normal range for a patient receiving 35 gtt/min of an IV containing 40,000 u heparin in 1 L D5W. The set calibration is a microdrip. _____

9. An IV of 35,000 u of heparin in 1 L D5W is ordered to infuse at 50 mL per hour. Calculate the hourly unit dosage. _____

10. A recent open heart patient has 500 mL D5W with 20,000 u of heparin infusing at 20 microdrips/min. Calculate the hourly unit dosage. _____

11. A physician orders a patient to receive 2000 u heparin IV hourly from a solution containing 50,000 u in 1000 mL D5NS. Determine the flow rate if the set calibration is 10 gtt/mL. _____

12. Order: Infuse a solution of 15,000 u heparin in 250 mL NS over 6 hours. Calculate the rate of flow if the set calibration is 20 gtt/mL. _____

13. A patient with a fractured pelvis has orders for an IV solution of 1 L D5 ½NS with 60,000 u of heparin. This is to infuse at 30 mL/hr. Calculate the hourly heparin dosage and determine if it is within normal range. _____

14. A physician orders a patient to receive 1000 u heparin IV hourly from a solution containing 20,000 u in 500 mL D5NS. Determine the flow rate if the set calibration is 60 gtt/mL. _____

15. A newly admitted patient has an order for IV heparin to infuse at 1500 u/hr continuously. The solution available is 20,000 u in 1 L D5W. The set calibration is 20 gtt/mL. Calculate the flow rate. _____

16. Calculate the hourly dosage of 1 L D5 ¼NS with 45,000 u heparin ordered to infuse at 25 mL/hr. _____

17. Calculate the hourly heparin dosage a patient with an IV of 40,000 u heparin in 1 L D5W infusing at 30 mL/hr is receiving. _____

18. A liter of solution containing 15,000 u of heparin is infusing IV at 20 gtt/min. Calculate the hourly unit dosage if the set calibration is 10 gtt/mL. _____

19. During morning rounds you time a patient's IV at 20 gtt/min. The solution infusing is 25,000 u heparin in 1 L D5W. The administration set delivers 10 gtt/mL. The doctor has ordered 1500 u of heparin per hour. Is the patient receiving the ordered dosage? _____

20. Order: Infuse 1 liter of D5RL with 25,000 u heparin over 24 hours. Using a set calibrated at 15 gtt/mL calculate first the hourly unit dosage then calculate the flow rate. Lastly determine if the dosage is within normal limits.

_____

21. A solution of 500 mL D5NS with 30,000 u heparin is infusing IV at 25 mL/hr. Calculate the hourly unit dosage and determine if it is within normal limits.

_____

22. For a patient with multiple fractures the doctor has ordered 2 liters D5 ½NS each with 20,000 u heparin to infuse at 50 mL per hour. Calculate the hourly unit dosage. The set calibration is a microdrip. What will the flow rate be?

_____

23. Calculate the mL/hr and hourly unit dosage for a patient receiving 500 mL D5W with 10,000 u heparin IV infusing at 20 gtt/min. Set calibration is 10 gtt/mL.

_____

24. Order: Infuse 1 liter D5W with 15,000 u heparin over 10 hours. Calculate mL/hr and u/hr being administered. _____

25. A patient is receiving 20 mL/hr of 1 liter D5W with 35,000 u of heparin. Calculate the hourly unit dosage and flow rate using a set calibration of 20 gtt/mL.

_____

ANSWERS

1. 40 gtt/min   **2.** 2250 u/hr   **3.** 34 mL/hr   **4.** 1600 u/hr   **5.** 25 mL/hr; 6 gtt/min   **6.** 11 gtt/min   **7.** 1042 u/hr; 7gtt/min
8. 1400 u/hr; Yes, within normal limits   **9.** 1750 u/hr   **10.** 800 u/hr   **11.** 7 gtt/min   **12.** 14 gtt/min   **13.** 1800 u/hr; No, dosage exceeds the normal range   **14.** 25 gtt/min   **15.** 25 gtt/min   **16.** 1125 u/hr   **17.** 1200 u/hr   **18.** 1800 u/hr   **19.** No, double the dose is infusing   **20.** 1042 u/hr; 11 gtt/min; Yes, dosage within normal limits.   **21.** 1500 u/hr; Yes, within normal limits
22. 1000 u/hr; 50 gtt/min   **23.** 120 mL/hr; 2400 u/hr   **24.** 100 mL/hr; 1500 u/hr   **25.** 700 u/hr; 7 gtt/min

25
Critical Care IV Calculations

OBJECTIVES
The student will calculate
1. dosages in mcg/kg per min/hr
2. dosages in mg per min/hr
3. IV flow rates in mL/hr
4. IV flow rates in gtt/min
5. discuss the use of electronic pumps in critical care
6. determine the tubing of choice in administering critical care drugs

INTRODUCTION
Physicians ordering critical care IV drugs generally order them by flow rate (**mL/hr, gtt/min**) or dosage, for example **mcg/kg/min or mg/hr**. It is necessary for you to learn how to calculate these minute but critical dosages and flow rates to better assess safe dosage ranges, and to monitor for any side effects or adverse reactions in drug response.

This chapter will cover methods of calculation to determine the dosage a patient is receiving per hour, per minute, per milliliter, and per drop. The patient's weight is also a critical factor in the ordered dosage, and it too is an important component of drug calculation.

Most critical care drugs require close and continuous monitoring. When available an electronic infusion pump should be utilized. Pumps have settings that allow solutions to infuse by mL/hr or gtt/min. Since these settings require calculations before administration, many of the problems in this chapter will ask you to determine the flow rate, either in mL/hr or gtt/min. In the event that an electronic pump is unavailable, select a tubing that delivers 60 gtt/mL, which is the next safest method of administration. These drops are very small, allowing greater control over incremental flow rate and dosage changes.

Remember, accuracy is imperative in calculating and administering critical care drugs because all have narrow margins of safety. Double checking math is both mandatory and routine.

Read each example and problem through first. Then go back and work through each step slowly and methodically. If you find yourself forgetting the steps you are moving too quickly.

• CALCULATING DOSAGE PER HR/PER MINUTE •

In critical care drug calculations always **determine the dosage first**. This will involve calculating the specific dosages per min and/or per hour. A drug may be ordered to infuse at a particular flow rate (mL/hr, or gtt/min) but remember to always determine the dosage first. To convert these flow rates to **dosage per hour or per minute**, the following steps are necessary.

EXAMPLE 1 Order: Infuse dopamine 800 mg in 500 mL D5W at 25 mL/hr. Calculate the dosage in mcg/min and mcg/hr.

- **Use ratio and proportion to determine the dosage per hour**

  800 mg : 500 mL = X mg : 25 mL

  800 × 25 = 500X

  20,000 ÷ 500 = X

  X = **40 mg/hr**

  The question asked the dosage in mcg/hr and mcg/min.

- **Convert milligrams to micrograms**

  40 mg = **40,000 mcg/hr** (move decimal three places to the right)

- **Convert mcg/hr to mcg/min**

  40,000 mcg/hr ÷ 60 min = **666.6 or 667 mcg/min**

EXAMPLE 2 A post-op cardiac bypass patient has orders to infuse Nipride at 30 gtt/min. The solution available is 100 mg Nipride in 500 mL D5W. Calculate the mg/min and mg/hr the patient is receiving. The set calibration is a microdrip.

- **First convert gtt/min to mL/min**

  60 gtt : 1 mL = 30 gtt : X mL

  60X ÷ 30 = **0.5 mL/min**

- **Calculate mg/min**

  100 mg : 500 mL = X mg : 0.5 mL

  100 × 0.5 = 500X

  50 ÷ 500 = X = **0.1 mg/min**

- **Calculate mg/hr**

  0.1 mg/min × 60 min = **6 mg/hr**

EXAMPLE 3 A patient with ventricular ectopi has stat orders for continuous Lidocaine infusion at a flow rate of 30 mL/hr. The solution available is 1 g Lidocaine in 500 mL D5W. Calculate first the mg/hr then the mg/min the patient will receive.

- **Convert the metric units in the stem of problem, (g) to the units asked for in the answer (mg)**

  1 g = 1000 mg

■ **Next determine the mg/hr**

1000 mg : 500 mL = X mg : 30 mL

30,000 ÷ 500X

X = **60 mg/hr**

■ **Convert mg/hr to mg/min**

60 mg/hr ÷ 60 min = **1 mg/min**

The average dosage of Lidocaine is 1–4 mg/min. From the answers you obtained you can quickly ascertain that the dosage is within a safe range.

EXAMPLE 4 0.5 g of Aminophylline is added to 500 mL D5 ¼NS. The order is to infuse IV over 6 hours. Calculate the mg/hr the patient will receive.

■ **Convert g to mg**

0.5 g = **500 mg**

■ **Calculate mg/hr**

500 mg : 6 hours = X mg : 1 hour

X = **83 mg/hr**

PROBLEM

1. A continuous infusion of Isuprel is ordered for a newly admitted patient in cardiogenic shock at 40 mL/hr. Solution available is 2 mg in 500 mL D5W. Calculate the mg/hr, mcg/hr, and mcg/min the patient will be receiving.

   _____

2. Order: Infuse dobutamine 500 mg in 500 mL D5W at 15 mL/hr. Calculate the mg/hr, mg/min, and mcg/min the patient is receiving.

   _____

3. Pronestyl 1 g in 250 mL D5W is ordered for a patient with frequent PVC's to run at 1 mL/min. Calculate the number of mg/min the patient is receiving. The normal dosage is between 2–6 mg/min. Is this dosage within normal limits?

   _____

4. A patient in CHF following an MI has an order for Nitrol IV 3 mL/hr by volumetric pump. The IV solution has a dilution of 200 mcg/mL of Nitrol. How many mcg/min and mcg/hr is the patient receiving?

   _____

5. Esmolol IV is ordered to control the ventricular rate of a patient during surgery. Solution available is 5 g in 500 mL D5W. The doctor orders the infusion to start at 50 mL/hr. Calculate the dosage in mg/hr and mg/min.

_____

6. To help support the blood pressure of a patient in shock, a doctor orders dobutamine 250 mg in 250 mL D5W to run at 25 mL/hr on a volumetric pump. Calculate the mg/min, mg/hr and mcg/min the patient is receiving.

_____

7. Order: Infuse dopamine 400 mg in 250 mL D5W at 30 gtt/min using a microdrip set. Calculate the mg/min and mg/hr the patient will receive. _____

_____

8. A doctor orders a Pitocin drip at 45 microdrops per min. The solution contains 20 u of Pitocin in 1000 mL D5W. Calculate the units per minute and the units per hour the patient is receiving. _____

9. 1 g of Aminophylline is added to 500 mL D5W. The order is to infuse IV over 10 hours. Calculate the mg/hr the patient will receive.

_____

10. Amikacin is ordered for a patient with a severe infection. Solution available is 500 mg in 250 mL D5W to infuse over 30 minutes using a volumetric pump. Calculate the mg/min the patient is receiving.

_____

ANSWERS **1.** 0.16 mg/hr; 160 mcg/hr; 2.7 mcg/min **2.** 15 mg/hr; 0.25 mg/min; 250 mcg/min **3.** Yes; 4 mg/min **4.** 600 mcg/hr; 10 mcg/min **5.** 500 mg/hr; 8 mg/min **6.** 25 mg/hr; 0.42 mg/min; 420 mcg/min **7.** 0.8 mg/min; 48 mg/hr **8.** 0.015 u/min; 0.9 u/hr **9.** 100 mg/hr **10.** 16.7 mg/min

Drugs are also ordered to infuse based on dosage per kg per min. For example, infuse 2 mcg/kg/min of a Nipride solution of 50 mg in 500 mL D5W. In this instance the first step is to determine the dosage per minute from the patient's body weight. Look at the examples below.

EXAMPLE 1 Order: 2 mcg/kg/min of Nipride
Solution available: 50 mg Nipride in 500 mL D5W
Patient's weight: 128 lb

■ **First convert lb to kg**

128 lb = **58 kg**

- **Calculate dosage per minute**

  58 kg × 2 mcg = **116 mcg/min**

  Infuse the Nipride solution at 116 mcg/min

EXAMPLE 2   Infuse a solution of 1 g Aminophylline in 1000 mL D5 ½NS at 0.7 mg/kg/hr. The patient weighs 169 lb. Calculate the dosage in mg/hr and mg/min. The drug literature states that you should not exceed 20 mg/min when infusing Aminophylline. Is this order within safe limits?

- **Convert lb to kg**

  169 lb = 77 kg

- **Calculate dosage per hour**

  77 kg × 0.7 mg = 54 mg/hr

- **Calculate the dosage per minute**

  54 mg/hr ÷ 60 minutes = **0.9 mg/min** Dosage is within safe limits.

EXAMPLE 3   A patient with Hodgkin's disease weighing 90 lb has orders for bleomycin sulfate 0.25 u/kg to be diluted in 50 mL of NS. Infuse over 30 minutes using a microdrip set. Calculate the dosage to be diluted then determine the u/min the patient will receive. This calculation involves only 1 additional step.

- **Convert lb to kg**

  90 lb = 41 kg

- **Calculate dosage to be diluted**

  41 kg × 0.25 u = **10.3 u** to be added to NS solution

- **Calculate dosage in u/min**

  10.3 u : 30 min = X u : 1 min

  10.3 ÷ 30 = **0.3 u/min**

PROBLEM

Calculate the drug dosage of the following orders.

1. A patient weighing 120 lb has orders for 6 mcg/kg/min of Nipride. Solution available is 50 mg in 250 mL D5W. Calculate the mcg/min and mg/hr.

2. A patient weighing 46 kg with testicular cancer has orders for Plicamycin 25 mcg/kg IV. The dosage is to be added to 1 liter of 0.9% NS and infused over 6 hours. Determine first the dosage you will prepare, then calculate the mcg/hr the patient will receive during the infusion. _____

3. Order: Give amphotericin B 1.5 mg/kg IV diluted in 500 mL D5W over 4 hours stat. The patient weighs 136 lb. Calculate the dosage you will prepare. Determine the mg/hr the patient will receive. _____

4. Infuse Nipride 2.5 mcg/kg/min. Solution available is 50 mg Nipride in 500 mL D5W. Patient weighs 62 kg. Calculate mcg/min and mg/hr. _____

5. A 70 kg adult has orders for a Lidocaine continuous infusion of 25 mcg/kg/min. Solution available is 500 mg Lidocaine in 250 mL D5W. Calculate the mcg/min and mg/hr. _____

ANSWERS   1. 330 mcg/min; 20 mg/hr   **2.** 1150 mcg; 192 mcg/hr   **3.** 93 mg; 23.3 mg/hr   **4.** 155 mcg/min; 9.3 mg/hr   **5.** 1750 mcg/min; 105 mg/hr

• CALCULATING IV FLOW RATES •

Once you have calculated the drug dosage the IV flow rate can then be determined. The flow rate is most often calculated in mL/hr or gtt/min as these are the most common methods of administration. Electronic pumps or controllers are the methods of choice in delivering these drugs but the specific flow rate needs to be determined before the machine is started. If an electronic device is unavailable, a microdrip set attached to a Buretrol may be your only alternative, but constant supervision of the drip rate is mandatory.

EXAMPLE 1   An ampule containing 400 mg of dopamine HCl is added to 500 mL D5NS. The order is to infuse 400 mcg/min IV. Using a volumetric pump calculate the flow rate in mL/hr.

■ **Determine the dosage per hour**

400 mcg/min × 60 min = **24000 mcg/hr**

■ **Convert mcg to mg (like units)**

24000 mcg/hr = **24 mg/hr**

■ **Calculate flow rate (mL/hr)**

400 mg : 500 mL = 24 mg : X mL
1200 = 400X
X = **30 mL/hr**

Set the flow rate at 30 mL/hr to deliver 24 mg/hr

EXAMPLE 2   A patient with severe chest pain has an order for a Nipride infusion. The order reads to add 50 mg Nipride to 500 mL D5W and infuse at 2 mcg/kg/min on a volumetric pump. The patient weighs 70 kg. Calculate the flow rate in mL/hr which will deliver this dosage.

■ **Determine the dosage per minute**

70 kg × 2 mcg/kg = **140 mcg/min**

■ **Convert to dosage per hour**

140 mcg/min × 60 min = **8400 mcg/hr**

The dosage per hour is necessary to calculate the flow rate (mL/hr).

■ **Convert to like units**

8400 mcg = 8.4 mg

■ **Calculate flow rate in mL/hr**

50 mg : 500 mL = 8.4 mg : X mL
500 × 8.4 = 50X
4200 ÷ 50 = X
X = **84 mL/hr**

Set the volumetric pump at 84 mL/hr to deliver 8.4 mg/hr

EXAMPLE 3   A patient in CHF has orders for Nitrostat 5 mcg/min IV. Solution available is 8 mg Nitrostat in 250 mL D5W. Calculate the flow rate in gtt/min using a microdrip set.

■ **Convert dosage per min to dosage per hour**

5 mcg/min × 60 min = **300 mcg/hr**

■ **Convert to like units**

300 mcg = **0.3 mg**

■ **Calculate mL/hr**

8 mg : 250 mL = 0.3 mg : X mL
X = 9.4 or **9 mL/hr**

■ **Calculate flow rate in gtt/min**

9 mL ÷ 1 (division factor) = **9 gtt/min**

To deliver 5 mcg/min set the flow rate at 9 gtt/min

PROBLEM

Calculate the following flow rates.

1. For a patient experiencing an acute MI with symptoms of shock, the doctor orders an infusion of Isuprel at 3 mcg/min. Isuprel 2 mg is added to 500 mL D5W. Calculate the mL/hr a volumetric pump would be set at to deliver this dosage.

   _____

2. Nitroglycerin 10 mcg/min is ordered to help sustain cardiac output. The solution strength available is 25 mcg/mL. Calculate the flow rate in gtt/min for an IVAC controller utilizing a tubing that delivers 60 gtt/mL. _____

3. A patient with ventricular irritability has orders to receive Pronestyl at 4 mg/min. Solution available is 500 mg Pronestyl in 250 mL D5W. Calculate the mL/hr the volumetric pump will deliver. _____

4. A Doxapram solution provides 20 mg/mL. Orders are to infuse at 3 mg/min IV. The set calibration is a microdrip. Calculate the correct flow rate in gtt/min.

   _____

5. A patient with angina has orders for a continuous IV infusion of Nitrostat. Solution available is 8 mg in 250 mL D5W. Orders are to infuse at 10 mcg/min. Calculate the flow rate in gtt/min using a microdrip. _____

ANSWERS **1.** 45 mL/hr **2.** 24 gtt/min **3.** 120 mL/hr **4.** 9 gtt/min **5.** 19 gtt/min

---

This concludes the chapter on critical care calculations most commonly encountered. The important points to remember from this chapter are:

- critical care drugs are generally ordered by dosage (mcg/kg/min, mg/hr), or by flow rate (mL/hr, gtt/min)

- always calculate the dosage first, double check your accuracy, then calculate the flow rate

- convert to like units whenever possible

- the safest method of administration is by an electronic device such as a volumetric pump or controller

- at any time electrical equipment can malfunction, so be prepared to monitor it routinely and check its accuracy

- ratio and proportion is still the safest and easiest method for calculating problems of this complexity

Critical Care IV Calculations

DIRECTIONS Read each question thoroughly then calculate only the dosages and flow rates indicated.

1. Dobutrex 6 mcg/kg/min is ordered to infuse IV to sustain the blood pressure of a patient weighing 165 lb. The solution available is 250 mg in 1 L of D5W. Calculate the mL/hr a volumetric pump will deliver. _____

2. Order: Infuse a Nipride solution of 50 mg in 500 mL D5W at 0.8 mcg/kg/min. Calculate the flow rate in mL/hr a 143 lb patient will receive. _____

3. A patient with aspiration pneumonia has an order for Aminophylline 1 g in 1000 mL D5W to infuse at 75 mL/hr. Calculate the dosage in mg/hr the patient will receive. _____

4. A solution of 400 mg dopamine HCl in 500 mL D5NS is infusing at 20 microdrops per min. Calculate the mg/hr the patient is receiving. _____

5. A doctor orders a pitocin drip by continuous IV infusion at 40 microdrops per min. The solution contains 20 u of pitocin in 1000 mL D5W. Calculate the hourly unit dosage. _____

6. A patient with bigeminy has orders to start an infusion of 500 mg Lidocaine in 250 mL D5W at 45 mL/hr. Calculate the mg/min and mg/hr this patient will receive. Is this within the normal range of 1–4 mg/min? _____

7. A terminal cancer patient has orders for continuous morphine sulfate IV. The solution available provides 0.5 mg/mL. The order is to infuse the drug at 8 mg/hr. Calculate the flow rate in mL/hr for a volumetric pump. _____

8. Order: Give 500 mg Aldomet in 150 mL D5W and infuse over 60 minutes. At what rate will you set the volumetric pump? _____

9. A patient in heart block has an Isuprel infusion ordered at 4 mcg/min. Solution available is 1 mg in 250 mL D5W. Calculate the flow rate in gtt/min for an IVAC controller. _____

10. For treatment of severe hypercalcemia a doctor orders Didronel 7.5 mg/kg diluted in 250 mL of NS to infuse over 3 hours. The patient weighs 101 lb. Calculate the dosage you would prepare, then determine the flow rate in mL/hour. Lastly, how many mg/hr would the patient receive? _____

11. 200 mg of dopamine is added to 250 mL D5W and an infusion is started at 45 gtt/min. Calculate the mcg/min and mg/hr the patient is receiving. _____

12. A patient with tetanus weighing 54 kg has orders for Thorazine 0.5 mg/kg in 500 mL NS. The infusion is run over 8 hours. First calculate the dosage, then the number of mL/hr at which you will infuse the drug. _____

13. A patient with chronic bronchitis and a severe respiratory infection is receiving 75 mL/hr of Aminophylline 1 g in 1 liter D5 ½NS. Determine the number of mg/hr the patient is receiving. _____

14. A physician orders 6 mg morphine sulfate every 30 minutes via a continuous IV drip. The available solution is 1 g in 1 liter D5NS. Calculate the flow rate in gtt/min using a microdrip. _____

15. A doctor orders 2 ampules of dopamine HCl to be added to 500 mL D5W to infuse at 25 mL/hr. Each ampule contains 200 mg. Calculate the mg/hr and mcg/min the patient is receiving. _____

16. A patient in CHF has orders to infuse 0.25 mg Lanoxin in 50 mL D5W over 15 min. Calculate the mg/min the patient will receive during the infusion.

    _____

17. Order: dopamine HCl 5 mcg/kg/min IV continuous. Solution available: 250 mL D5W with 400 mg dopamine. Patient weight is 155 lb. Calculate the flow rate in mL/hr for a volumetric pump. _____

18. The doctor orders Pronestyl 3 mg/min IV. Solution available 500 mg in 250 mL D5 ¼NS. Calculate the flow rate in mL/hr. _____

19. A nitroglycerin solution of 25 mcg/mL is infusing at 30 gtt/min. Calculate the mcg/min the patient is receiving. _____

20. A patient with aplastic anemia has orders for 5 g Amicar to be added to 250 mL NS and infused over 90 min. Calculate the mg/hr and flow rate in gtt/min using a microdrip set. _____

21. Order: give 7 mg/kg of Amikin IV in 250 mL D5W over 2 hours. Patient weighs 180 lb. Calculate the dosage you would prepare then the mL/hr to deliver the drug on time. _____

22. For treatment of a gram negative infection the doctor has ordered polymyxin B 12,000 u in 500 mL D5W at 200 mL/hr. Calculate the u/hr the patient is receiving. _____

23. A patient with severe hypotension is receiving 3 mL/min of a solution of Levophed that contains 4 mg in 500 mL D5W. Calculate the mcg/min the patient is receiving. _____

24. A continuous infusion of Aminophylline at 0.7 mg/kg/hr is ordered for a patient weighing 98 lb. Solution available is 1 g in 1 liter D5W. Calculate mL/hr for delivery on a volumetric pump. _____

25. A patient in hypertensive crisis has orders for Arfonad 1.5 mg/min IV. Solution available is 500 mg in 500 mL D5W. Calculate gtt/min using an IVAC controller.

    _____

ANSWERS

1. 108 mL/hr   2. 31 mL/hr   3. 75 mg/hr   4. 16 mg/hr   5. 0.8 u/hr   6. 1.5 mg/min; 90 mg/hr; Yes   7. 16 mL/hr   8. 150 mL/hr
9. 60 gtt/min   10. 345 mg; 83 mL/hr; 115 mg/hr   11. 36 mg/hr; 600 mcg/min   12. 27 mg; 63 mL/hr   13. 75 mg/hr   14. 12 gtt/min
15. 20 mg/hr; 333 mcg/min   16. 0.017 mg/hr   17. 13 mL/hr   18. 90 mL/hr   19. 13 mcg/min   20. 3,333 mg/hr; 167 gtt/min
21. 574 mg; 125 mL/hr   22. 4800 u/hr   23. 24 mcg/min   24. 32 mL/hr   25. 90 gtt/min

INDEX